# Overcoming Isometrics

Text Copyright © 2020 Matthew John Schifferle
All Rights Reserved

# ISBN- 9798639077517

The information provided in this book is designed to provide helpful information on the subjects discussed. This book is not meant to be used, nor should it be used, to diagnose or treat any medical condition. For diagnosis or treatment of any medical problem, consult your physician. The publisher and author are not responsible for any specific health or allergy needs that may require medical supervision and are not liable for any damages or negative consequences from any treatment, action, application or preparation, to any person reading or following the information in this book. References are provided for informational purposes only and do not constitute an endorsement of any websites or other sources. Readers should be aware that the websites listed in this book may change.

The scanning, uploading, and distribution of this book without permission is a theft of the author's intellectual property. If you would like permission to use material from the book (other than for review purposes), please contact Matt Schifferle at Reddeltaproject@gmail.com. Thank you for your support of the author's rights.

Cover photo and design by Chris Clemens at
http://www.thinkpilgrim.com

Dedicated to the Red Delta Project Community.

Thank you for all of your support and inspiration.

# Table Of Contents

Intro: Your Best Workouts Are Still Ahead of You    5

1 How to Enhance Every Workout You'll Ever Do    11

2 Extension Chain Isometrics    29

3 Push Chain Isometrics    37

4 Pull Chain Isometrics    46

5 Squat Chain Isometrics    57

6 Flexion Chain Isometrics    63

7 Lateral Chain Isometrics    73

8 Hybrid Isometrics    80

9 Training Strategies for Success    90

10 Tools of the Trade    97

11 Frequently Asked Questions    101

# Your Best Workouts Are Still Ahead Of You

The simple techniques and methods in this book will help you take your current workouts to the next level and beyond.

If you're new to exercise, this book will help you quickly establish a rock-solid foundation to build you up to your ultimate potential. If you're a seasoned athlete, these same methods will infuse new life and vigor into any workouts or exercises that have grown stale. These methods have been in use for centuries, yet you'll only need to apply these techniques for a few weeks to notice an improvement in how you look, feel and perform.

If that sounds good to you, then you've come to the right place.

**Your yet-to-be-discovered potential**

Mother Nature has bestowed upon your muscles with an unbelievable amount of adaptive power. Eons of evolution have hard-wired your muscles with the potential to make you far more capable than you may currently believe. The trick is in finding a way to recognize and tap into that primal transformative potential.

Ever since the first warriors and acrobats started training, people have been trying to figure out how to unleash their ultimate physical power. In ancient times, physical conditioning was especially crucial for warriors and hunters whose physical abilities meant the difference between life and death.

Eventually, the discipline of conditioning the body spread beyond the niche interests of athletes and fighters. Now, everyone from sedentary executives to busy homemakers are joining gyms and working out in the pursuit of health and physical transformation.

As the interest in physical change has grown, so have the attempts to sell products to assist in such change. Sadly, many of these products and services have left earnest, hard-working folks, just like yourself, still wanting to get more from their training. We now live in a world that's filled with hype and promises, yet short on satisfying results.

Our modern fitness culture has created an interesting paradox. On the one hand, we now have more knowledge and resources to get in shape than in any other time in human history. On the other hand, successful physical transformations are an incredibly uncommon occurrence. They are so rare that you often have to turn to social media, instead of real life, to find examples of impressive and inspiring physiques. Look up from your phone, while at the gym during rush hour, and tell me how many people there look even half that good. You probably won't find many such examples.

**Why is that lazy idiot jacked, and I'm not?**

There are, of course, those few outliers who hold our attention because they are the .01% who've built a fantastic physique. What's more, they often seem to make it look as if it's the most natural thing in the world. Meanwhile, the rest of us have to work twice as hard for a fraction of the progress. It just seems so unfair!

It's easy to make excuses for why only a few can achieve such success. Many will point their finger at steroids and lucky genetics to account for the large discrepancy between the haves and the have-nots. Unshakeable discipline and an obsessive work ethic are also influences for sure. Those factors are undoubtedly important, but I've discovered that there's a lot more to the story. I know this because I'm one of those lucky bastards who's built an uncommonly impressive physique with seemingly little effort. At least that's been the case for the part of my physique between my feet and knees.

You see, I've been sporting a rather impressive set of calves ever since my late teens. My lower legs are my most complimented body part by far. I've even had competitive bodybuilders pull me aside in the gym and ask me what my secret is.

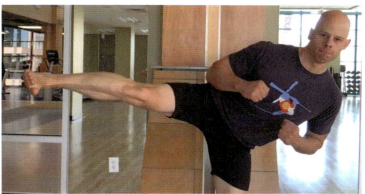

*My calves have long been one of my most aesthetically strong features despite hardly ever working them directly.*

The honest answer is, I don't do very much for my calves. Sure, I hit a few random sets of standing calf raises once in a while, and I'm an avid cyclist, but I understand those are hardly satisfying answers.

There are countless examples of people doing calf raises and pushing pedals, yet they can't seem to grow their calves even a little. That's why I'm never surprised when people claim my calves are the result of luck and good genetics. It only makes sense, especially when you consider the fact that the calves are one of the most stubborn muscle groups to grow.

The truth is, I have long held a special calf training secret; only it was so secret that even I didn't know I possessed it. And no, it's not just genetics. (Although genes do play their role in the overall shape of the muscle.) It's a secret that's so subliminal, yet powerful, that it can make or break your muscle building success regardless of any other factors.

**The all-powerful importance of neuro-muscular proficiency**

In my last book, Grind-Style Calisthenics, I mentioned that something called neuro-muscular proficiency is the ultimate foundation of effective physical training.

Neuromuscular proficiency is the general term for how well you can engage and use your muscles through mental concentration. The skill of mental muscle activation controls everything from how strong you can contract a given muscle to your muscle endurance, coordination, and even stability. To put it simply, if your neuromuscular proficiency is high, then your workouts are going to be far more productive no matter what sort of routine or program you're following. Unfortunately, if your neuromuscular proficiency is lacking, you can work as hard as possible with the best methods in the world; and still not get very far.

Neuromuscular proficiency is one of the biggest reasons why there are such impressive physical outliers in our fitness culture. Look into the history of anyone with an impressive physique, and you'll undoubtedly discover they learned how to master the use of their muscles early in their career. Maybe they started working out with their state-champion powerlifting dad when they were a kid. Perhaps they took an interest in gymnastics or joined the high school Olympic lifting team. Whatever the case, someone along the way taught them how to use their muscles effectively. That neuromuscular education gave them a considerable advantage every single day of their training career.

That was certainly the case with my calves. When I was younger, I asked a friend how he could jump so high in our Taekwon-Do class. He told me, "it's all in the toes," and he showed me how to hop around on the balls of my feet by using my calf muscles. From that point on, I ran, hiked, biked, and even walked on the balls of my feet.

All of this calf-dominant movement built up a powerful neural connection between my brain and my lower legs. By the time I was bike racing in college, my calves were the most dominant muscle group in my entire body. Every step and pedal stroke would send a tidal wave of muscle tension through my calves, which made them grow like weeds.

It took me about 10 years to develop my awareness of neuromuscular proficiency. Once I became aware of it, its influence was very obvious everywhere I looked. I started to develop a sixth sense for identifying where clients had a strong or weak neural drive just from how their physique looked or how they moved. If anyone had an underdeveloped area of their body, it was a sure-fire bet they were lacking neuromuscular proficiency in that area.

Discovering my lack of neuromuscular proficiency helped me learn why one of my most stubborn muscle groups refused to grow. I always seemed cursed to have small and narrow shoulders. All of the lateral raises and shoulder presses didn't help in the least bit, and now I know why. When I started lifting, I suffered some chronic shoulder pain, especially in my right shoulder. Eventually, I had to see a physical therapist to break up the scar tissue that had built up in my shoulders. I was able to get back to a pain-free state, but the neuromuscular proficiency in my shoulders never recovered. This weakness has been more than enough to seriously handicap my upper body and shoulder development.

Thankfully, the techniques in this book have helped me turn the tide, and I'm finally building up my shoulders for the first time in my training career.

Discovering the power of neuromuscular proficiency has been the single most significant discovery I've made in my training career and the training of my clients. It is, without a doubt, the essential factor in any form of successful training. The only question now is, how exactly does someone improve their neuromuscular proficiency?

That single question is why I've written this book detailing the fastest and easiest strategy to improve your neuromuscular proficiency. Your best workouts are still out there, and this book will help you discover them and the incredible transformative power they hold.

# 1

# How to Enhance Every Workout You'll Ever Do

Learning about the importance of neuro-muscular proficiency is one thing; figuring out how to improve it is an entirely different kettle of fish. People have been experimenting with ways to enhance their neuromuscular ability for centuries with various levels of success. You can find some of the most ancient methods in old disciplines like Yoga, Qi-gong, and martial arts. Old-time strongmen like Charles Atlas and Maxick created whole training methods based on techniques to improve neuromuscular proficiency.

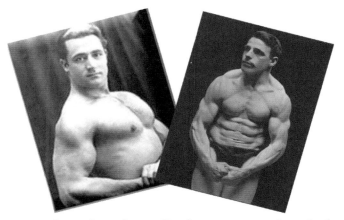

*Maxick was a true pioneer in understanding how to create and manipulate muscle tension for building strength.*

In more recent times, strength training with free weights and machines have become a popular choice.

All of these methods work to some degree; however, they also all have a few disadvantages that can hold you back. It's these disadvantages that have created such a hit-or-miss rate of success within our modern fitness culture.

So let's take a look at precisely what neuromuscular proficiency is, and how you can quickly enhance it for lasting results.

**Building a bigger engine**

I like to use the analogy of a sports car when explaining the importance of training your nervous system for physical improvement. In a car, the most attention-grabbing parts are the wheels. After all, the wheels are where the actual rubber meets the road. However, if you want to make a car go faster and perform well, you know that it's not the actual wheels that make the car move. Instead, it's the engine and transmission that provides the power to the wheels, which then transfers that mechanical energy into movement.

When it comes to the human body, it's easy to place too much attention on the muscles. There's a lot of information out there about muscle fibers, muscle growth, and even protein to feed the muscles.

This information is useful, but you may be neglecting the actual internal engine that's truly responsible for your physical ability. Your real strength doesn't originate in your muscles, but rather your nervous system. When it comes to driving your body, it's your brain and nervous system that's sending instructions to your muscles.

It's easy to fall into the trap of believing that your muscles work because of the exercise you do, or the weight you lift. While the dumbbell in your hand is an influence on the resistance on your body, it's not physically making your muscles contract. The instructions to lift the weight are coming straight from your brain and nervous system.

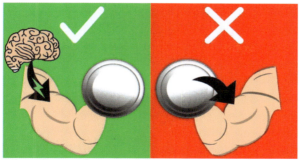

*Muscle tension doesn't come from a weight or even an exercise; it comes from your mental focus and concentration.*

Also, if you look at a high-end sports car, you'll notice the wheels are super sporty and lightweight. They will even be wearing a set of low-profile slick racing tires too. Those wheels and tires look cool, but they don't make the car go fast. Instead, they are there so the driver can better handle the power coming from the engine.

Your muscles work the same way. They don't get bigger and stronger just because of the exercise you do or the equipment you use. That would be like me driving my Honda Civic on a race track to make my wheels look like the wheels on a Ferrari. Instead, your muscular wheels adapt to the power coming from your neural engine. When you upgrade your neural drive, you force your muscles to adapt to handle that force. However, your muscles will never adapt if you continue to drive the same amount of neural power to them no matter what you do in your workouts.

## The four parts of neuromuscular proficiency

Building a bigger neural engine is the most critical thing you can do in the pursuit of building bigger and stronger muscles. But before we get into exactly how to do that, let's look at the four parts that make your neural engine work.

# #1
# NEURAL CONNECTION

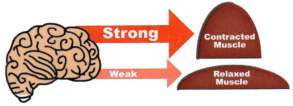

Your neural connection is the ultimate foundation of your neuromuscular proficiency and, therefore, the effectiveness of every exercise you do. Your neural connection is also one of the biggest reasons why many people struggle to strengthen a given muscle group. If your brain has trouble sending a signal to a muscle, you simply cannot work it effectively.

Some of the most common areas that suffer from a poor neural connection are the abs, hips, hamstrings, and all of the muscles in the back. Most of this is due to our ingrained habit of sitting so much. The less you use a given muscle, the more the neural pathway between your mind and muscle atrophies. Luckily, the opposite is also the case as the more you use a neural pathway, the stronger that connection becomes.

# #2
# NEURAL SYNERGY

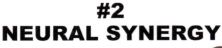

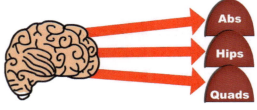

Neural synergy is your ability to simultaneously engage multiple muscle groups and use them in a coordinated way. This synergy helps reduce stress in your joints while also making it possible to move with grace and skill. You've undoubtedly experienced this anytime you've tried to learn a sport or physical skill.

When it comes to building muscle and strength, neural synergy is crucially important. The coordinated use of muscle tension helps create physical stability while also allowing the stress of an exercise to flow safely through your body. Without those two things, you'll have unstable joints, which will make you weaker and more prone to injury.

## #3
## NEURAL STRENGTH

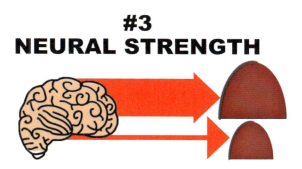

Neural strength is the actual strength of the signal your brain is sending to your muscles. The stronger that signal is, the more muscle fibers you engage at a given time, and the harder you contract the muscle. Simply put, a stronger neural signal builds a bigger and stronger muscle.

## #4
## NEURAL ENDURANCE

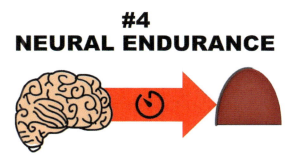

Your neural endurance refers to the amount of time you can continue to send the signals to your muscles so you can force them to continue to work.

This type of endurance is much more than just the physical stamina of your muscles themselves. A lot of your actual endurance is mental stamina, and how long your mind can concentrate on sending a strong signal to your muscles.

I've witnessed the power of neural stamina many times when someone suddenly discovers the ability to perform more reps due to a mental trick. One of my favorites is to perform an exercise as long as possible without counting reps. When someone tells me they can only do so many push-ups, I ask them to do a set but not to count the reps. Most of the time, they blow right past their old rep limit and keep going. It's not a Jedi mind trick; it's because they've grown accustomed to doing a certain number of reps so their mind would start shutting off the neural signal as they continued to count. Without counting the reps, their mind didn't have a numerical reference point, so it didn't know when it was supposed to turn down the neural signal.

Neural endurance is also a crucial factor in building muscle. An effective muscle building workout often requires pushing your muscles to a high level of fatigue, which is only possible with a high degree of neural endurance. You can have a lot of neural strength to make a muscle very strong, but making that muscle work hard for an extended period is the key to growth.

**Building a more powerful neural engine**

All four parts of this neural engine work together in a coordinated way, just like the parts of an actual engine. Let's use deep bodyweight squats to illustrate how this is the case.

The first part, neural connection, is crucial because you simply cannot go into a deep squat if your mind has difficulty engaging specific muscles. One of the most common examples is a lack of neural drive to the hamstrings and hip muscles, which help pull your hips down and forward into the bottom position.

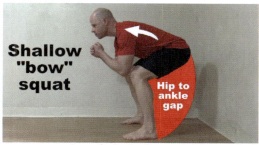

*A shallow squat is a common sign of a lack of neural drive to the hamstrings and hip muscles.*

Once you have a neural connection to your lower body muscles, you can improve your neural synergy to make all of the individual muscles work together as one complete unit. Not only will the neural synergy progress your ability to squat lower, but you'll also have less stress on your joints and feel more stable in the bottom position.

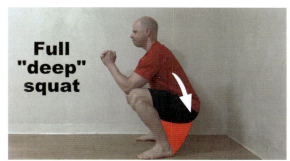

*A strong neural connection to the muscles in the back of your legs is the key to accomplishing a deep squat.*

The next part, neural strength, is then built off of the foundation of your neural synergy. Your mind can only create a strong neural signal in a stable environment. If you've ever tried to run on ice or do push-ups with a sore shoulder, then you know exactly how this feels.

When you feel unsafe and unstable, your mind will naturally put on the neural brakes and refuse to send a strong signal to your muscles. Therefore, improving your neural synergy will create a more stable environment, which then promotes a much stronger neural signal.

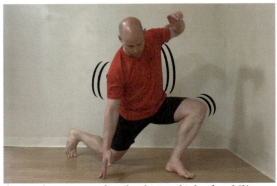

*A lack of neural synergy often leads to a lack of stability and balance.*

Lastly, creating a robust neural signal is the foundation of neural endurance. The stronger and more confident you feel, the longer your mind will be able to create a lasting signal. However, when you lack strength, your mind will become overwhelmed with even a modest amount of work and fatigue very quickly.

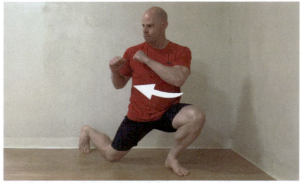

*Neural synergy is the key to full-body stability even while moving in multiple planes of motion.*

Each level of this neural hierarchy builds onto the foundation of the layers beneath it. A stronger neural connection will promote neural synergy. Better neural synergy will develop more neural strength, and more neural strength will foster far more neural endurance. If you want to build muscle, you need to have good neural stamina.

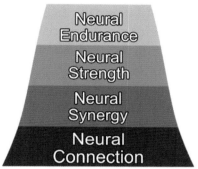

*The neural hierarchy helps you understand the foundation of physical ability and development.*

**Why working out sometimes doesn't work out**

Despite popular belief, working out doesn't always have the best track record of helping people get the results they want. If anything, success in the gym is the exception rather than the norm.
Observing the neuromuscular proficiency hierarchy is one of the keys to solving the mystery behind why some people struggle to get results despite pushing themselves hard with proven workout programs.

Working out, even very hard, is not a very reliable way to improve your neuromuscular proficiency. Sure, exercise *might* improve your neuromuscular proficiency for a little while, but this improvement is usually pretty limited to a few weeks. After that, you hit a seemingly endless plateau no matter how hard you work or what sort of program you use.

It's not the fault of the exercise or the workout program. It's our own fault for assuming that our body will somehow automatically know how to control the tension in our muscles. This assumption is a dangerous one to make because all types of strength training can potentially fail to address one or more of the four aspects of neuromuscular proficiency.

For example, strength training that focuses too much on low rep training can fail to adequately develop your neural stamina. At the same time, too much high rep training can fail to sufficiently improve your neural strength. Single joint strength training is one of the best ways to strengthen the neural connection to a given muscle group. That's why such focused exercises are prevalent in restorative practices like physical therapy. The downside is that too much attention to isolated movements can hinder your neural synergy since you're not practicing how to use your muscles in a coordinated way.

Compound movements can be great for improving your neural synergy, but again, that's assuming you have a strong neural connection to every muscle that should be involved in the exercise. If one of those muscles has a weak connection, your mind will create a very efficient, and often subliminal, compensation pattern to work around that muscle so you can still perform the activity, albeit to a lower level of technical quality.

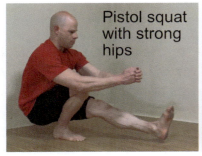
Pistol squat with strong hips

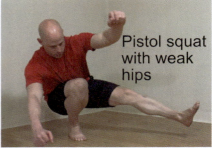
Pistol squat with weak hips

It's worth noting that no amount of hard-core training will ever fix a lack of neural connections, synergy, strength, or stamina. The longer and harder you train, the more you reinforce your old neuromuscular habits. Eventually, these imbalances can lead to injury, poor performance, stiffness, and a general sense of ill-ease about the body.

The common knee-jerk reaction is to blame the exercise or program you were using during the injury, but this is a misguided attempt to fix the problem. Chances are, the exercise or program isn't causing the problem so much as it's exposing the real issue. If you only avoid the troublesome activity, you're still bringing the same neural imbalances to whatever else you attempt to do next, and the problem only gets worse.

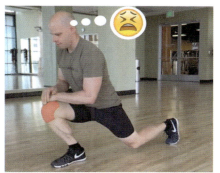 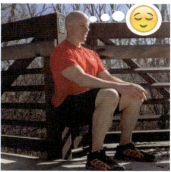

*Avoiding lunges because they make your knees sore can offer some temporary relief, but it doesn't address the real problem at hand which may be a lack of tension control in the hamstrings.*

## The ultimate neural hack for effective workouts

Okay, enough of the doom and gloom talk. It's time to stop focusing on the problems that may be holding you back and start learning about an easy, simple, and very effective solution called *overcoming isometrics.*

Isometric training is any physical discipline that involves keeping your body in the same position. So instead of counting movements or reps, like with dynamic exercise, isometric training is done for time as you hold a given position.

You may be more familiar with what is known as *yielding isometrics*, where you hold your body in a position against a set level of resistance. Some of the most common examples include typical core work, like planks and L-sits or handstands.

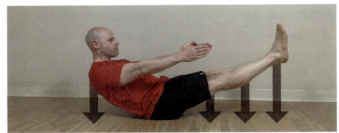

*The hollow body hold is a classic yielding isometric exercise where you hold yourself in position against the pull of gravity.*

Yielding isometric training can be a useful discipline; however, it causes you to relate to a source of resistance (in this case, gravity) in much the same way you would with classic dynamic exercises. As such, it can be quite difficult to avoid any subliminal neural compensation habits. Yielding isometrics are a great strength and muscle building tool, but can still fall short of being a proper neural training tool.

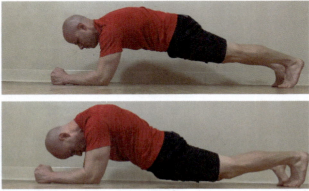

*You may be able to hold a yielding isometric for a long time, but what's happening to the quality of your technique to make that happen?*

Overcoming isometrics is unique in the fact that you don't work against an external source of resistance like gravity or resistance bands. Instead, you apply force against an immovable object, which creates resistance directly proportional to your muscle tension. This scenario creates the perfect environment for developing optimal neuromuscular proficiency.

**The overcoming isometrics advantage for training your neural connection**

The primary objective for most exercises is to accomplish the act of doing the exercise. Again, this is primarily due to the assumption that the mind automatically knows how to best use your muscles in order to accomplish the task at hand.

Nevertheless, the theory is that you'll get the results you want if you just do the right exercises, lift the right weight, or follow the right program. Therefore, the objective of each rep, set, and workout quickly becomes about doing the work as opposed to how well you're using your muscles. This assumption can be easy to make, but even the best workout won't produce the results you want if you lack neuromuscular proficiency.

The legendary tension control pioneer, Maxick understood this concept all too well in his book Muscle Control.

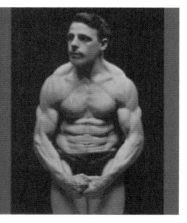

"Mechanical exercise will only produce good results if interest is directed to the muscles being used. If the mind is directed only to work being performed, a certain point of muscular resistance is reached; but there it stops. To secure full benefit from the exercise it is essential that the mind be concentrated on the muscles, and not the work performed."

These days, it's very fashionable to just perform the activity with as much effort as possible instead of considering technical proficiency. The idea is that anyone can achieve excellent results if they are only willing to work hard enough. Different people measure their effort in different ways. Some people strive to lift as much weight as they can, or perform as many reps as possible. Others use speed and a quick pace to jack up their heart rate and work up a good sweat.

A hard effort is essential to your success, but results are contingent upon having a decent amount of neuromuscular proficiency while you apply that effort.

If your neuromuscular proficiency is lacking, you may be doing more harm than good since a high degree of effort and intensity can reinforce dysfunctional neuromuscular habits. The harder you push, the more you reinforce your bad habits and muscle imbalances. This ingrained neural compensation is often why some people experience a jump in their results when they back off on their workout intensity and lift a bit lighter, cut back on volume, or slow down their pace.

Overcoming isometrics avoids all of this potential compensation because the objective isn't to hit some ego-driven metric or to be satisfied with merely wearing yourself out. Instead, the focus of every overcoming isometric exercise is to improve how well you can engage and use your muscles at will. This seemingly small difference in mental focus can make a very large difference in steering your strength training into more productive territory.

**The overcoming isometrics advantage for training your neural synergy**

It's almost impossible to ignore weaknesses and neural compensation with overcoming isometrics. The exercises in this book are like a massive spotlight that shouts, "OVER HERE! HERE'S SOMETHING YOU NEED TO TAKE CARE OF!"

Not only will such weaknesses become very apparent, but you'll naturally start to address those weaknesses through practicing basic overcoming isometric exercises.

This advantage is why overcoming isometrics can be the ultimate neural assessment and diagnostic tool for muscle imbalances and improving your neural synergy.

**The overcoming isometrics advantage for training your neural strength**

I used to believe it was impossible to build a decent amount of strength with techniques that didn't involve any movement. I reasoned that contracting a muscle was what created a movement, therefore movement = strength. I now know I was very much mistaken in this regard. If anything, the best methods for building pure strength are the ones that involve less movement, not more.

The reason for this is due to something called the force-velocity principle in physiology. The basic idea is that the more tension you put in a muscle, the slower you move. This principle is why excessive tension in a muscle can be detrimental in sports that require a lot of speed like sprinting or punching. On the other hand, high-strength activities like powerlifting use a very slow rate of speed due to the high degree of muscle tension that's required to lift such impressive amounts of weight.

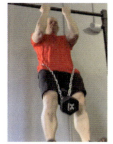 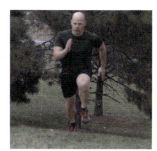

*The more tension you generate, the slower you move. Running up a hill is slower than running on flat ground or lifting a heavier weight makes you slower than lifting a lighter one.*

So the formula is simple, if you want to challenge your strength, you'll need to use methods that don't allow you to move at a high rate of speed.

The slower you have to move, the more tension you'll have in the muscle. Naturally, the slowest speed you can move at is not to move at all, which is the case with isometric training. Once you eliminate the need to move through space, you remove the limitation of how much tension you can put into a muscle. You're free to contract your muscles as hard as you possibly can, which puts you on the fast lane to conditioning your neural strength.

As a side bonus, overcoming isometrics is also a very safe and comfortable way to create that level of tension. It can take a lot of time and practice to be able to safely and effectively develop near-maximum levels of tension with large amounts of weight.

Overcoming isometrics makes it much more comfortable, and safer for even rank beginners to push their muscles as hard as possible due to the lack of movement and external load.

**The overcoming isometrics advantage for neural endurance**

Movement can also be a hindrance to developing your neuromuscular endurance. Once again, this is due to the force-velocity principle.

All physical movement requires at least some degree of strength, and you can only continue to perform a motion as long as your muscles can produce enough tension to do so. Once your muscles become too fatigued, you have to stop practicing the movement. The dichotomy between strength and endurance is why it's difficult to train simultaneously for strength and endurance. The more strength you use, the less time you can perform the exercise. If you want to perform an exercise for an extended period, you'll have to back off how much tension you're using in your muscles.

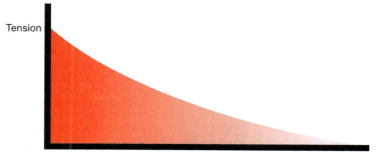

Overcoming isometrics doesn't require movement, which means you'll never reach a state of muscular failure where you have to discontinue an exercise. You can now work your muscles very hard while also maintaining tension for long periods thus allowing you to work on generating maximum tension and maximum endurance at the same time.

All four of these advantages add up to make overcoming isometrics one hell of a neural training powerhouse. It's a simple and highly efficient training method that automatically adjusts to your exact level of fitness and present physical condition. It seamlessly optimizes your neural connection, synergy, strength, and stamina all at the same time. Couple those advantages to the fact that you can train overcoming isometric exercises every day, and you have a method for quickly creating a significant amount of progress.

When you look at it, overcoming isometrics may very well be the single most efficient training method in existence. Nothing else requires so little time, skill, energy, effort, or equipment while also providing such a wide range of benefits. It almost seems crazy *not* to do them.

So let's start to get your hands dirty and explore some of these simple and efficient exercises.

# 2

# Extension Chain Isometric Exercises

Your extension chain includes all of the muscles along the backside of your body. The major muscle groups include your calves, hamstrings, glutes, lower back, and spinal erectors.

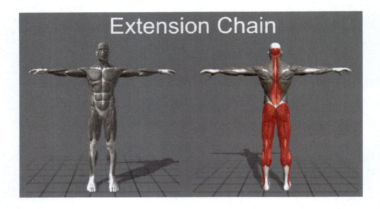

If there's one area of the body that can stand to benefit the most from overcoming isometrics, it's most certainly the extension chain. This group of muscles contributes a significant influence on every movement you practice. It also includes your glutes and hamstrings, which are the powerhouse for many athletic activities.

Unfortunately, the extension chain is also one of the biggest neural wastelands due to modern sedentary habits, like sitting. Most everyone suffers from poor neural connection, synergy, strength, and stamina to some degree in their extension chain. These imbalances leave the door wide open for potential injuries and poor performance.

To make matters worse, many of the modern strength training methods are making the situation worse rather than better. Most modern weight machines usually involve doing the exercises from a seated position, which only amplifies the neural patterns of sedentary habits.

Even weight machines that attempt to remedy the issue, like the "lower back machine," only emphasize tension in one area of the chain. This attempt to isolate the work into the lower back only further inhibits the neural synergy between the upper and lower halves of the chain.

In recent years, ground-based free weight training has become more popular with the proliferation of kettlebells, Olympic lifting, and deadlifting. All of these movements should be an absolute blessing to the extension chain since they require a lot of neural strength, endurance, and synergy along the extension chain. Unfortunately, handing someone a heavy barbell or kettlebell is just like giving a teenager the keys to a Ferrari. Ground-based exercises are only safe and effective once you can first assess, and build, the neural proficiency necessary to execute those techniques safely and effectively.

Thankfully, the following overcoming isometric exercises will do wonders to reverse the detrimental effects of sedentary living while priming your neural proficiency.

# Standing Hip Extension

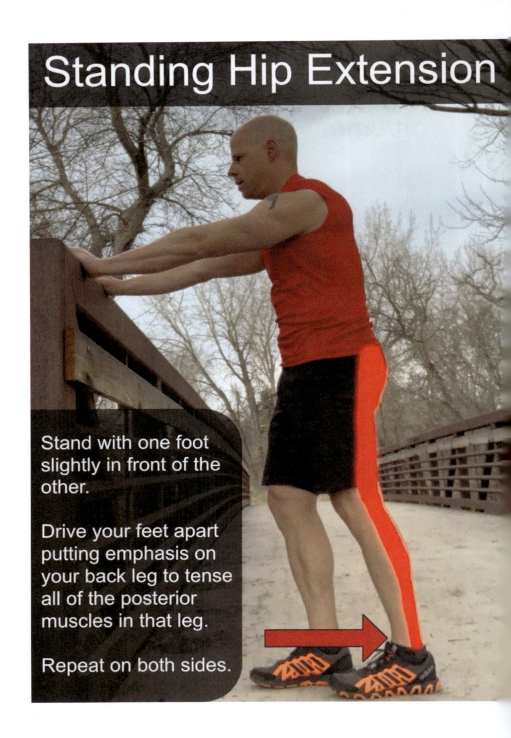

Stand with one foot slightly in front of the other.

Drive your feet apart putting emphasis on your back leg to tense all of the posterior muscles in that leg.

Repeat on both sides.

# Lying Hamstring Curl

Lay down on the ground with your feet on the ground and your knees bent at a 90 degree angle.

Drive your heels into the ground to lift your hips up with your glutes and hamstrings.

Pull your heels backward into the ground to squeeze the ground between your shoulders and feet.

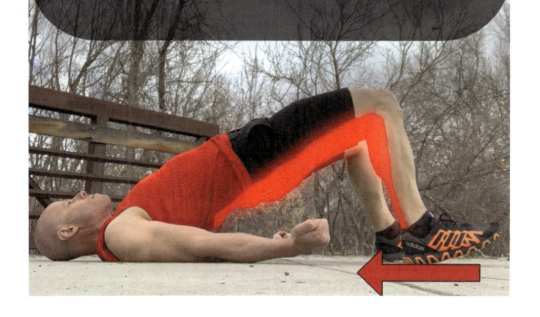

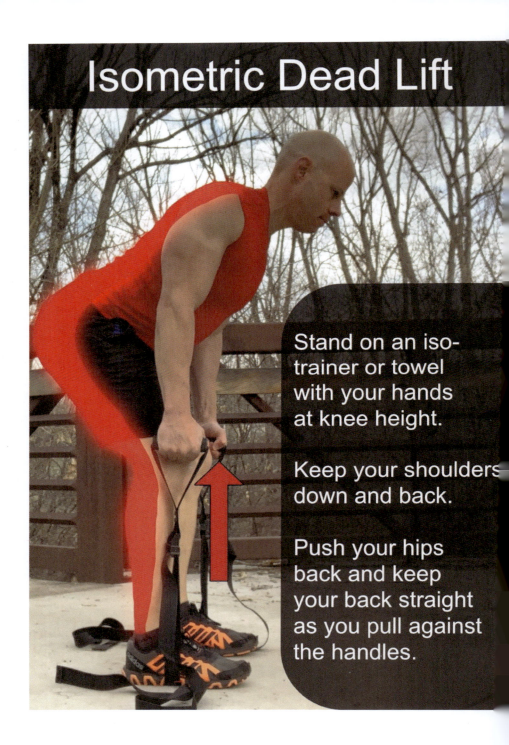

# Table Bridge

Sit on the ground and place your hands slightly behind your hips with your arms straight.

Drive your heels into the ground with your knees bent 90-degrees to lift your hips into "table" position.

Use your hamstring to pull your heels back toward your hands.

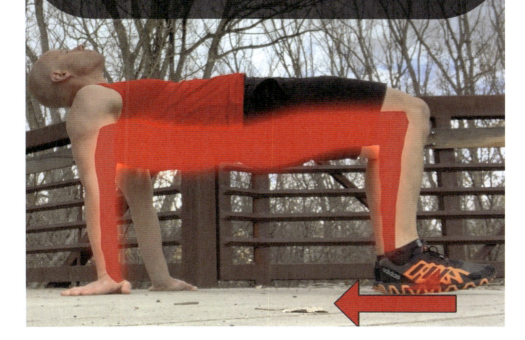

# Calf Raise

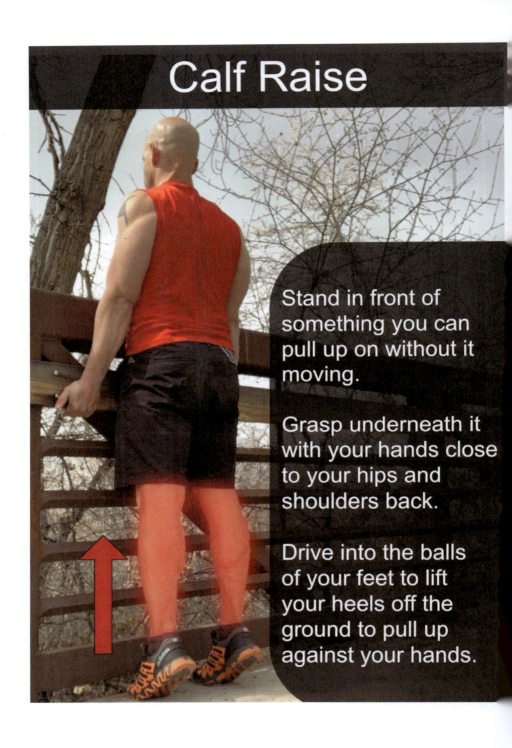

Stand in front of something you can pull up on without it moving.

Grasp underneath it with your hands close to your hips and shoulders back.

Drive into the balls of your feet to lift your heels off the ground to pull up against your hands.

# Rear Neck Extension

Wrap an iso-trainer or towel around the back of your head.

Hold your hands in front of your face while keeping your neck straight.

Pull your head back against your hands while applying forward pressure with your hands.

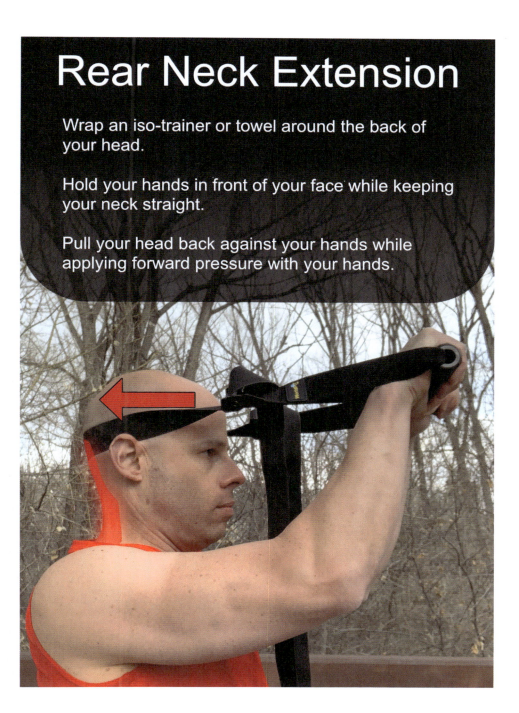

# 3

# Push Chain Isometric Exercises

The push chain is one of the most popular muscle groups to work, especially when you consider the popularity of exercises like push-ups, handstands, dips, bench presses, and any activity involving lifting weight overhead. This chain includes all of the muscles in your chest, shoulders, triceps, and forearm extensors.

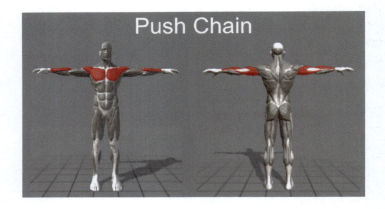

Due to its popularity, it's easy to assume that the neural proficiency of the push chain must be relatively high for most people, but this is seldom the case. Remember that neuromuscular proficiency is a skill and like any skill, there's no guarantee that endless hours of practice will polish it to perfection. Practice only reinforces your neural habits. It doesn't guarantee the proficiency of the habits you need to succeed.

Such neural reinforcement is why many athletes find they have trouble building their chest and triceps despite years of hard training. They can camp out on the bench press all day long and do push-ups until they are peeling themselves off the floor all they like. All of that hard work won't guarantee a bigger chest or broader shoulders if they have trouble engaging those muscles from the onset.

Thankfully, the following exercises will help you quickly develop neuromuscular proficiency in your push chain and significantly improve the quality of your pressing exercises.

# Standing Chest Press

Wrap an Iso-trainer or yoga strap around your shoulders and press your hands forward.

Keep your shoulders back and elbows in to maximize tension in your chest and triceps.

Be sure not to shrug your shoulders upward, but keep them down away from your ears.

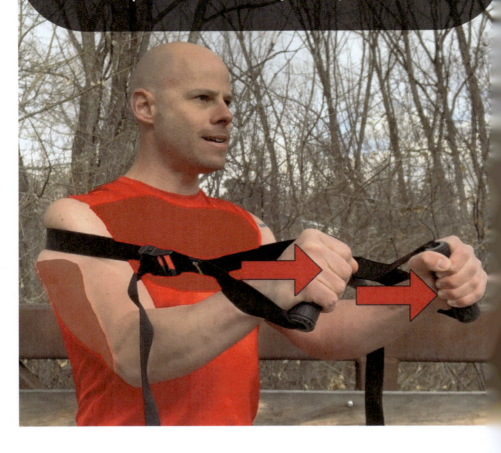

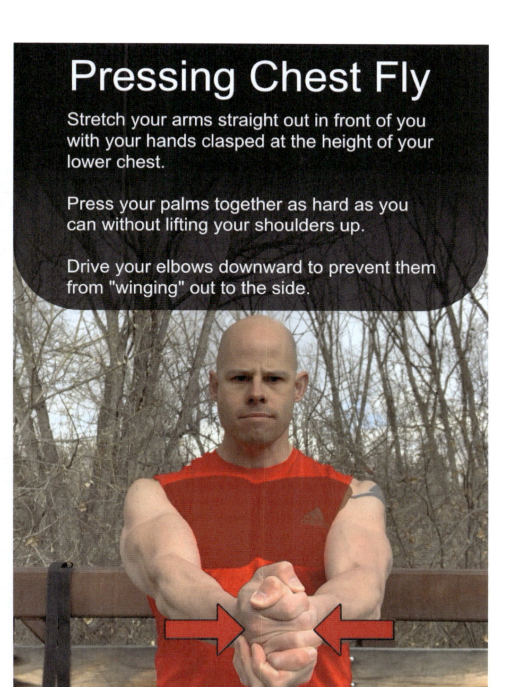

# Standing Overhead Press

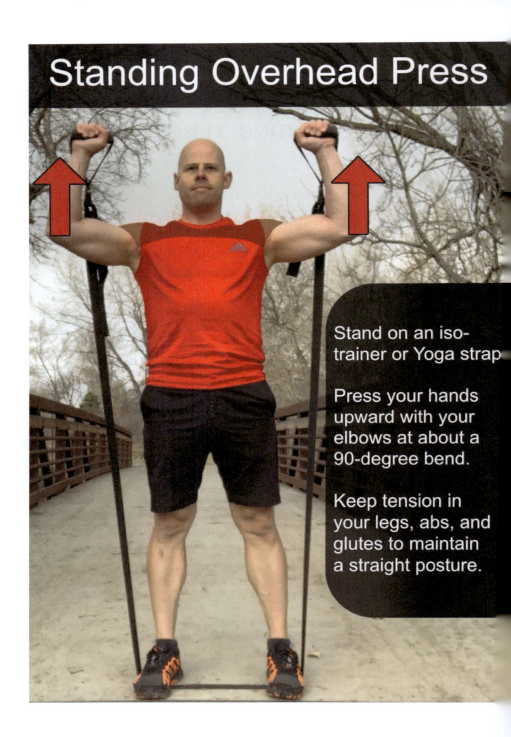

Stand on an iso-trainer or Yoga strap

Press your hands upward with your elbows at about a 90-degree bend.

Keep tension in your legs, abs, and glutes to maintain a straight posture.

# Standing Shoulder Raise

Stand on an Iso-trainer or Yoga strap and pull your arms upward while keeping them straight.

Position your arms at a slight downward angle.

Experiment with holding your arms more to your front or side to see where you can feel it best.

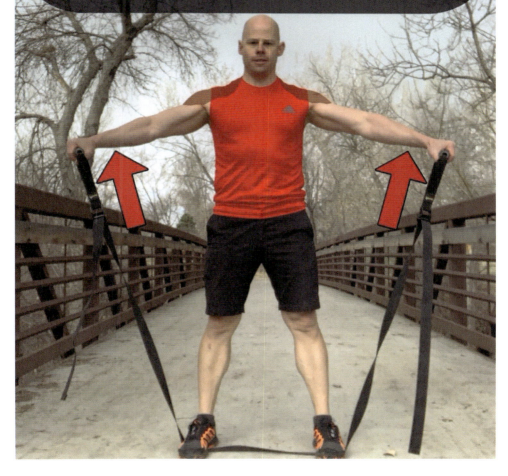

# Lateral Shoulder Raise

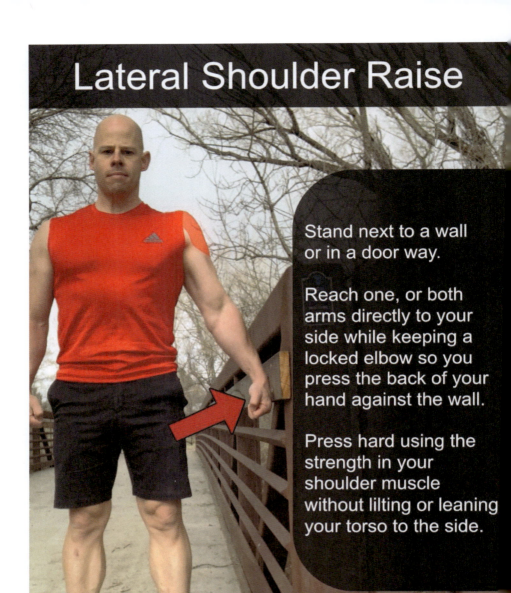

Stand next to a wall or in a door way.

Reach one, or both arms directly to your side while keeping a locked elbow so you press the back of your hand against the wall.

Press hard using the strength in your shoulder muscle without lifting or leaning your torso to the side.

# Triceps Push-Down

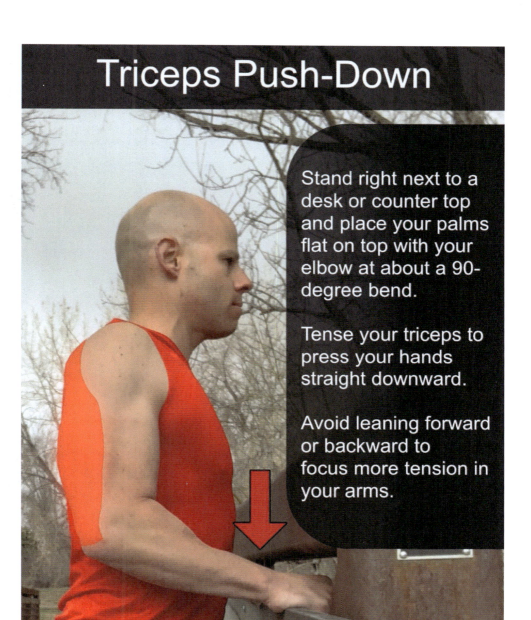

Stand right next to a desk or counter top and place your palms flat on top with your elbow at about a 90-degree bend.

Tense your triceps to press your hands straight downward.

Avoid leaning forward or backward to focus more tension in your arms.

# Wrist Extensions

Extend your arms, either in front of you or down by your sides.

Straighten your fingers and pull them back as if you're trying to touch the top of your fingers to your forearm.

Try to get all of your fingers to pull back evenly.

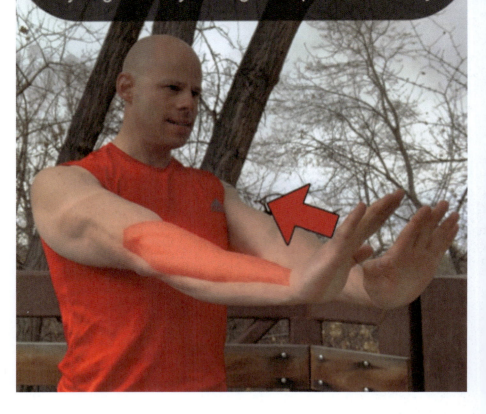

# 4

# Pull Chain Isometric Exercises

Your pull chain includes all the muscles in your back, including your traps, latissimus dorsi, and shoulder muscles like the Infraspinatus. Your pull chain also contains the pulling muscles in your arms like your biceps, brachialis, and forearm flexors.

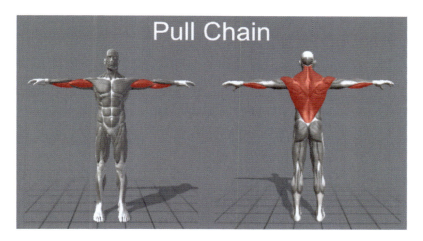

You use this tension chain with all exercises that involve pulling your hands closer to your torso, like rows and pull-ups, as well as yielding isometric techniques like hanging and carrying. While it does include some of the biggest and strongest muscles in your upper body, it's also one of the most fragmented tension chains for many people.

One of the most common forms of tension fragmentation is when people have a reliable connection to muscles, like the biceps and lats, but have a weak neutral connection with their upper back and shoulders. Another variation is having a strong neural connection with the upper back and grip, but poor tension control in the lats.

In either case, this neural fragmentation usually leads to less overall strength and power along the pull chain and underdeveloped muscle groups. This neural fragmentation is also one of the leading causes of stress in the joints with golfers or tennis elbow being common injuries, especially for those who practice a lot of pull-ups.

As always, doing more exercise and knocking out high-rep workouts isn't a viable solution for such neural fragmentation. Add in high-resistance exercises like weighted pull-ups or heavy dumbbell rows with poor neural synergy, and you have a recipe for disaster. Thankfully, the following overcoming pulling exercises will quickly remedy any imbalances and weaknesses to build a super strong and resilient pull chain.

# Seated Row

Sit on the ground with a strap or towel around your feet and your arms at a 90 degree angle.

Set you shoulders down and back while squeezing your arms in tight to your sides.

Pull hard on the strap while ensuring you keep tension in your forearms and biceps.

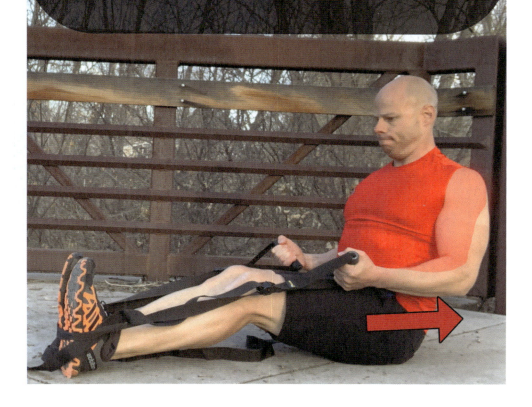

# One-Arm Seated Row

Sit on the ground with a strap or towel around your feet and hold the other end with one hand.

Pack the shoulder of your working arm down and back with a slight twist in your torso.

Drive your elbow back as hard as possible while keeping tension in your bicep and forearm.

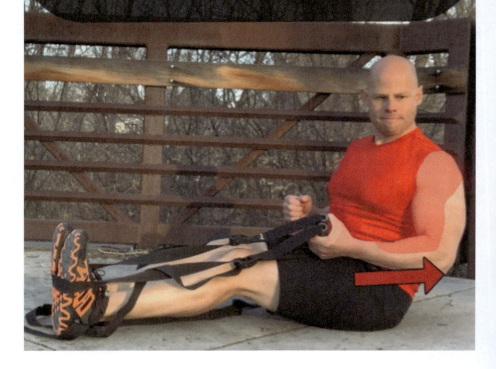

# Lying Elbow-Press Row

Lay flat on the ground with your shoulders down while pinching your shoulder blades with your elbows bent at a 90 degree angle.

Squeeze your arms in tight to your side.

Drive your elbows into the ground while also pressing down into the back of your heels to maintain tension along your extension chain. You should feel all of the muscles on your backside working, not just your traps and lats.

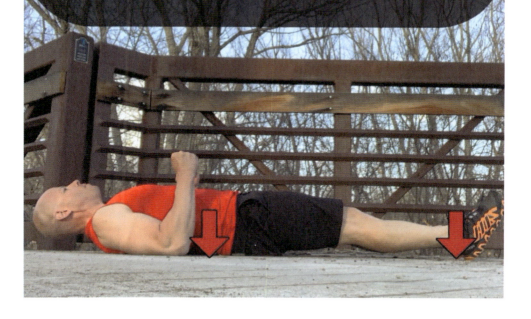

# Rear Fly

Sit on the ground with a strap or towel over your feet.

Pull your hands back while keeping your arms straight and down at a slight angle.

Focus on using all of the muscles in your upper back while pinching your shoulder blades together.

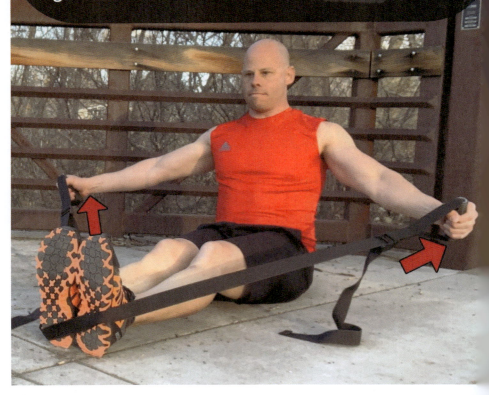

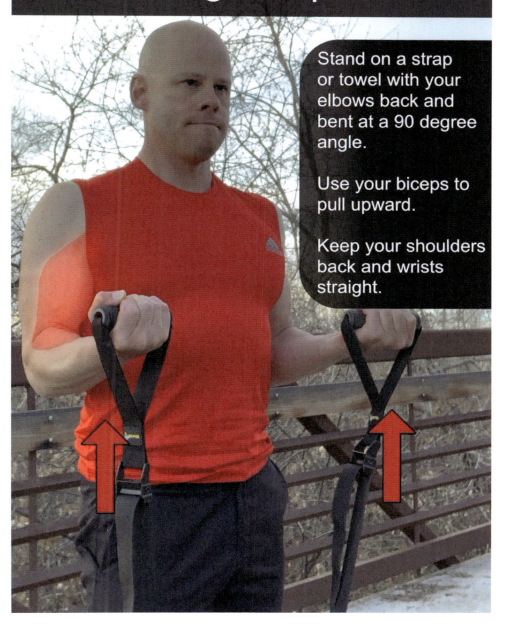

# Standing Lat. Squeeze

Stand on a strap or towel and hinge your hips back with your knees slightly bent.

Drive your hands back while keeping your arms straight while Squeezing your arms into your sides.

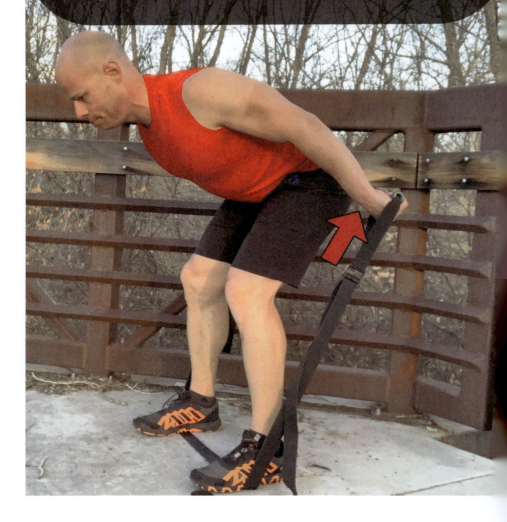

# External Shoulder Rotation

Grip a strap or towel with your elbows bent at a 90 degree angle.

Pull your hands apart while keeping your elbows close to your ribs and your shoulders down and back.

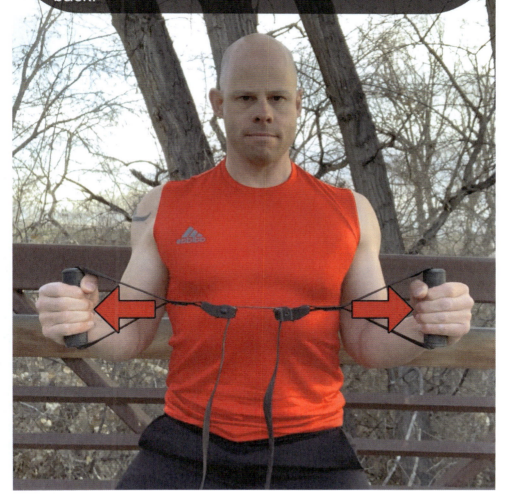

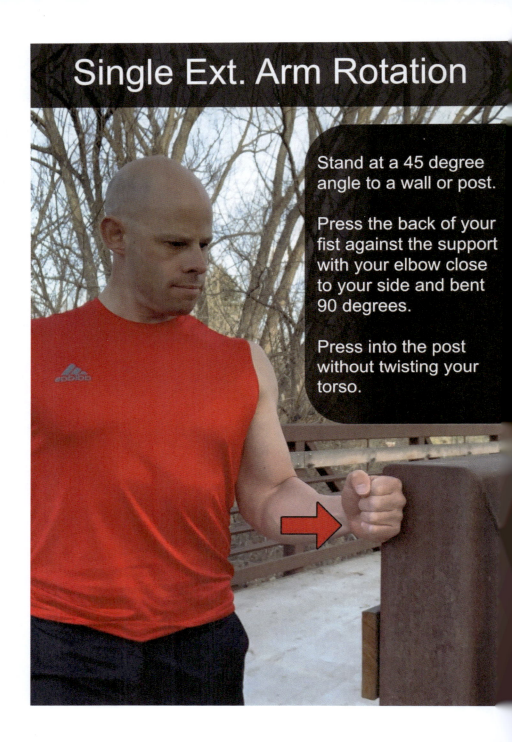

# Wrist Flexion

Straighten your arms either in front of you or let your arms hang down by your sides.

Clench your hands into loose fists.

Curl your fists down as if you're trying to touch your thumbs to your forearms.

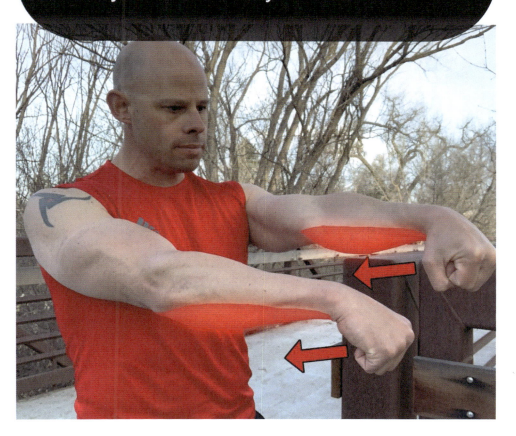

# 5

# Squat Chain Isometric Exercises

Your squat chain includes your quads and hamstrings, as well as your glutes and hip muscles. Finally, you have the muscles in your lower leg, including your calves and the muscles in your shins.

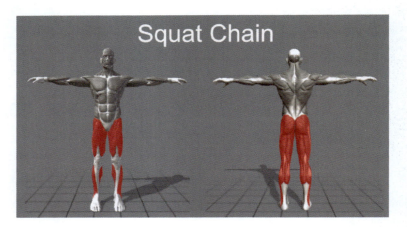

As the name implies, your squat chain is involved with any squatting motion where you change the distance between your hips and ankles. Naturally, this includes the primary leg strengthening exercises like squats and lunges, but it also consists of all other lower body activities like walking, running, stepping up, cycling, and jumping.

You'll notice the back-side of your legs also includes the muscles from your extension chain. This observation points out why the same neural fragmentation that's common with the extension chain can also influence your squat chain.

Some of the primary areas of neural weakness are the hips and hamstrings. However, unlike the extension chain, the squat chain also helps to resolve issues relating to the front and lateral hip muscles. This holistic approach to lower body tension is the key to creating a strong pair of legs.

It's also worth noting that the following overcoming isometrics may help you with any instability and strength plateaus you may be experiencing with dynamic lower body exercises. This is because most lower body training only briefly transitions you through the bottom position of your squats and lunges. While dynamic leg work is very effective, few people spend enough time in a crouched position, which challenges the strength and stability of the lower body. Don't be surprised if you find your muscles working pretty hard the first time you're trying out these techniques, especially if you're not used to holding the bottom of a squat or lunge.

# Front Squats

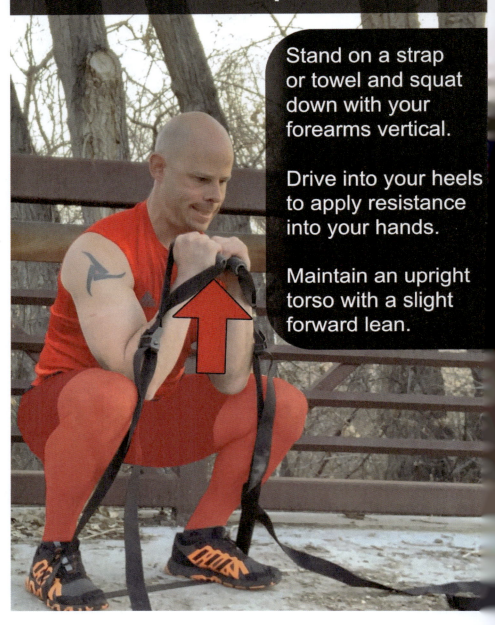

Stand on a strap or towel and squat down with your forearms vertical.

Drive into your heels to apply resistance into your hands.

Maintain an upright torso with a slight forward lean.

# Front Lunges

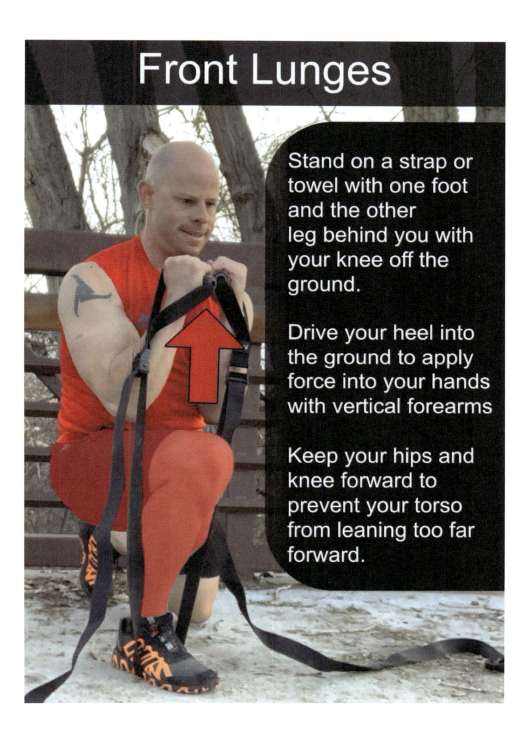

Stand on a strap or towel with one foot and the other leg behind you with your knee off the ground.

Drive your heel into the ground to apply force into your hands with vertical forearms

Keep your hips and knee forward to prevent your torso from leaning too far forward.

# Zercher Lunge/ Squat

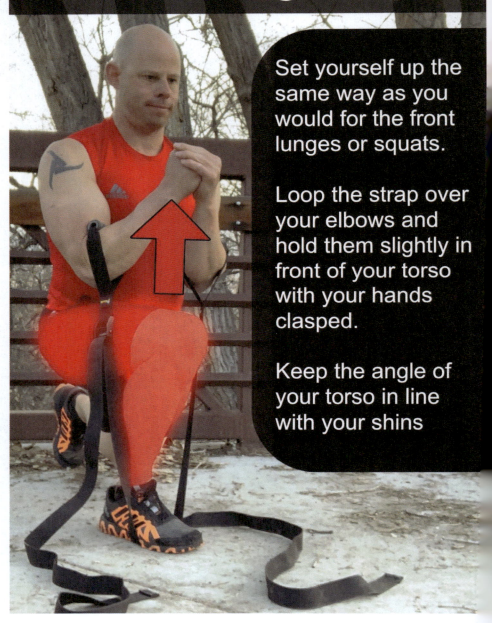

Set yourself up the same way as you would for the front lunges or squats.

Loop the strap over your elbows and hold them slightly in front of your torso with your hands clasped.

Keep the angle of your torso in line with your shins

# Wall Leg Extension

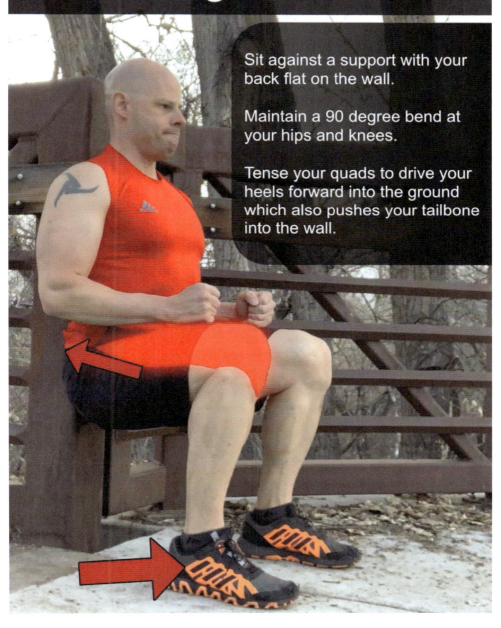

Sit against a support with your back flat on the wall.

Maintain a 90 degree bend at your hips and knees.

Tense your quads to drive your heels forward into the ground which also pushes your tailbone into the wall.

# 6

# Flexion Chain Isometric Exercises

Your flexion chain uses all of the muscles along the front of your body. This tension chain includes the front of your neck, abs, hip flexors, quads, and even the muscles in your shins.

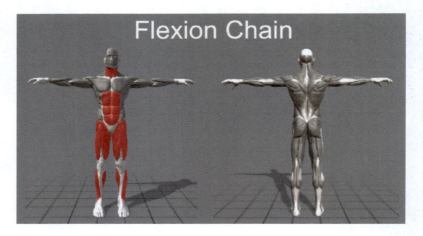

If there's any muscle group that can stand to gain a lot from overcoming isometrics, it's the abs. Chronic neural deconditioning is a pervasive issue for many people, even among the most gifted athletes and dedicated exercise enthusiasts.

The prevalence of weak flexion chain neuromuscular proficiency is a curious thing when you consider just how much time and attention people often place on core training. As a trainer, the midsection is by far the most popular area people tell me they want to exercise. There are also scores of gadgets, books, classes, and YouTube videos all about ab training and how to achieve that coveted six-pack. You would think that all of this attention to one area of the body would produce astonishing results, but that's very rarely the case.

Very few people get very far in their abdominal pursuits despite all of the attention they give to that area of their body. The proliferation of all of those products is just further proof that most of the conventional approaches don't work very well. If they did, there wouldn't be very much unsatisfied demand driving the creation and distribution of such products.

As you may guess, a big reason why so many people struggle to achieve their six-pack goals is that they suffer from poor neural proficiency. You can use the latest equipment and apply the most cutting edge workouts all you like, but it will hardly make any difference if you can't get your abs to turn on in the first place.

The good news is that the opposite is also the case. Once you improve the neural proficiency of your core muscles, anything you do will become vastly more productive. So without further ado, let's explore some of the most effective overcoming isometrics for your abs and the flexion tension chain.

# "Cat" Floor Squeeze

Kneel down with your thighs and arms perpendicular to the floor.

Tuck your pelvis up into a posterior tilt to crunch your abs and create a slight arch in your lower back.

Contract your abs to squeeze the floor together between your hands and knees.

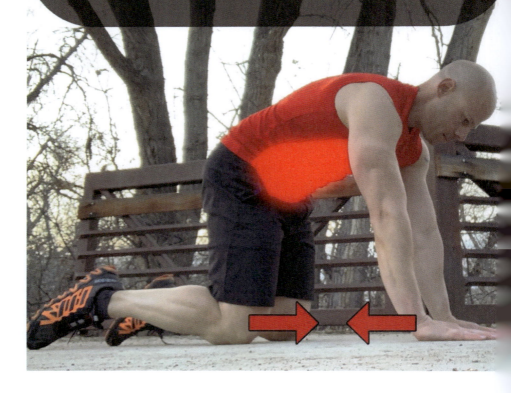

# Plank Floor Squeeze

Get into a hollow body straight arm plank position with your hips tucked into a posterior pelvic tilt.

Use your abs to try to squeeze the floor together between your hands and feet.

Ensure you keep your weight equally balanced between your hands and feet.

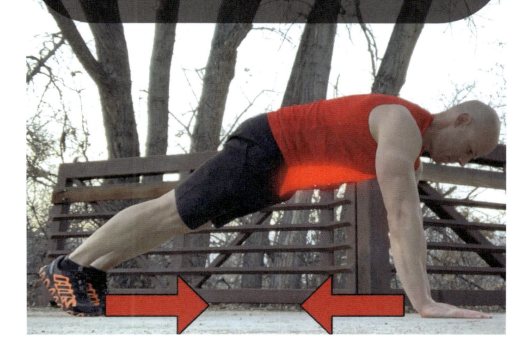

# Dead Bug

Lay on the ground and pull your knees up close to your chest.

Crunch your abs to lift your shoulders off the ground and press your hands or forearms into your knees.

Contract your abs to drive your hands and knees together as hard as you can.

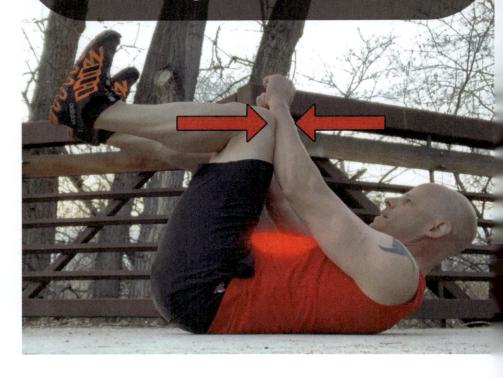

# Abdominal Pull-Down

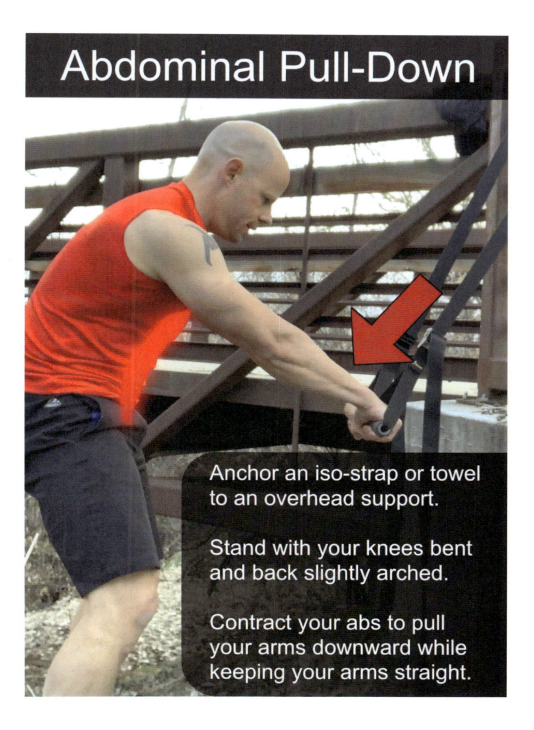

Anchor an iso-strap or towel to an overhead support.

Stand with your knees bent and back slightly arched.

Contract your abs to pull your arms downward while keeping your arms straight.

# Oblique Pull and Twist

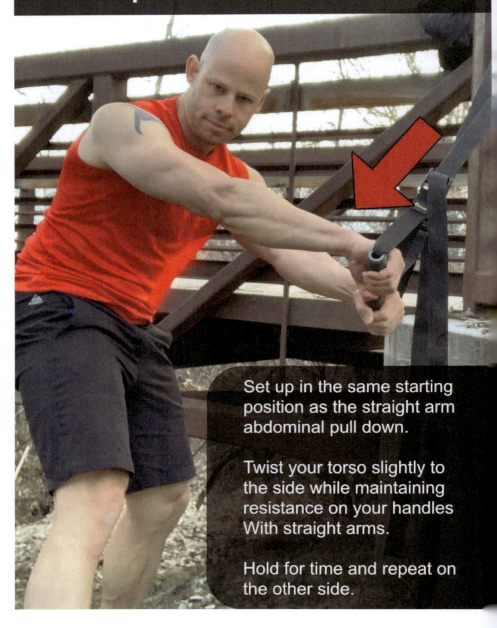

Set up in the same starting position as the straight arm abdominal pull down.

Twist your torso slightly to the side while maintaining resistance on your handles With straight arms.

Hold for time and repeat on the other side.

# Duck Walk

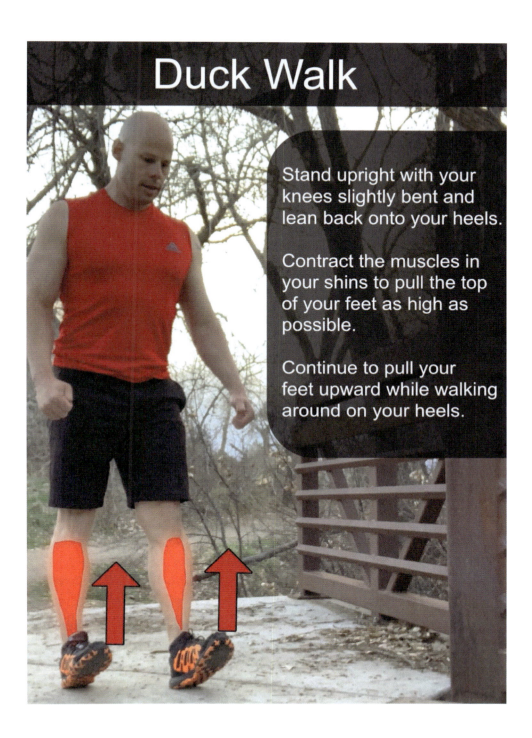

Stand upright with your knees slightly bent and lean back onto your heels.

Contract the muscles in your shins to pull the top of your feet as high as possible.

Continue to pull your feet upward while walking around on your heels.

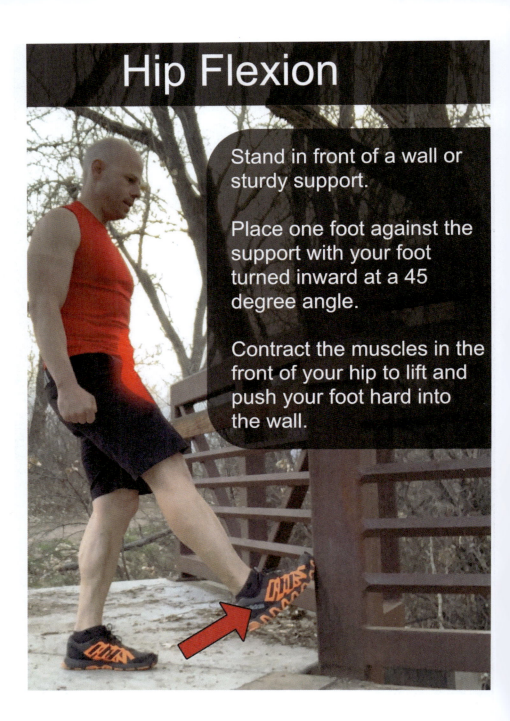

# Hip Flexion

Stand in front of a wall or sturdy support.

Place one foot against the support with your foot turned inward at a 45 degree angle.

Contract the muscles in the front of your hip to lift and push your foot hard into the wall.

# Neck Flexion

Sit on a sturdy seat with the back of your elbows on your knees and your forehead against your palms.

Tense your abs and neck muscles to press your forehead into your hands.

Try to keep your neck in line with your spine

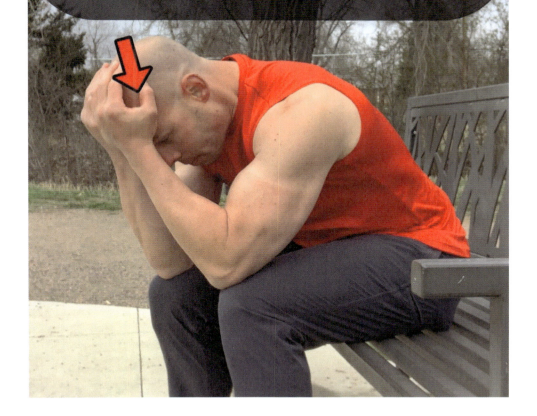

# 7

# Lateral Chain Isometric Exercises

The lateral chain is yet another chain that stands to reap a lot of benefits from overcoming isometrics. Not only is this area often considered part of the "core," which is often neurologically weak, but also because the lateral chain plays a unique role in total body strength and performance.

Your lateral chain works sort of like the glue that helps all of your other tension chains connect and work together so your body can function as a whole unit.

Your lateral chain includes the muscles along each side of your body. These include your lateral hamstrings, quads, inner and outer hips, obliques, spinal erectors, lats, shoulders, and neck.

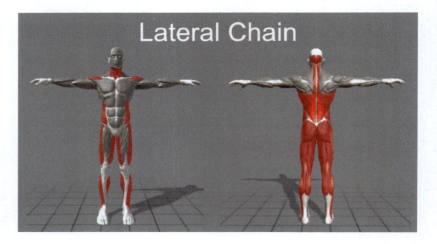

You'll probably notice that you use these muscles with several other tension chains. This inclusion is why these groupings aren't really about specific muscle groups so much as they are the use of tension along with those muscles. It's for this reason why training your lateral chain is so important. You'll still be using all of those muscles with other exercises, but none of the techniques so far make the whole side of your body operate as one cohesive unit.

Learning how to engage and create neural synergy along the full sides of your body is extremely important in all aspects of strength and performance; these exercises will help you do just that.

# Lateral Press Down

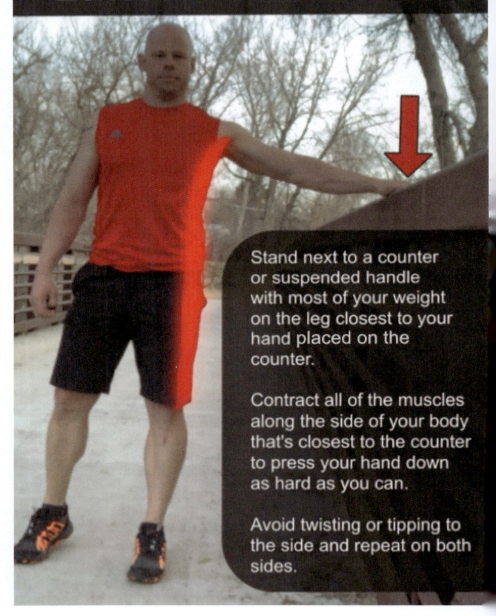

Stand next to a counter or suspended handle with most of your weight on the leg closest to your hand placed on the counter.

Contract all of the muscles along the side of your body that's closest to the counter to press your hand down as hard as you can.

Avoid twisting or tipping to the side and repeat on both sides.

# Squeezing Side Plank

Lay down on the floor in a classic side plank position with your shoulder back and your shoulder, hips and feet in a straight line.

Keep your shoulders back as you squeeze the floor together between your feet and supporting forearm.

Do your best to drive your bottom foot straight into the floor to maximize tension in your hips.

Repeat on both sides.

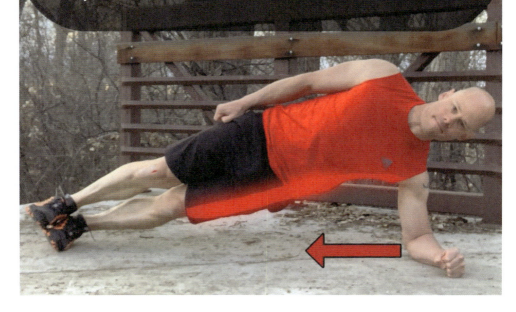

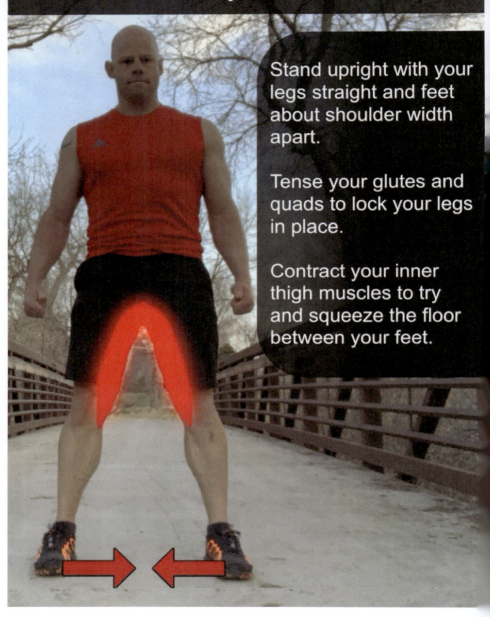

# Lateral Hip Adduction

Stand upright with your legs straight and feet about shoulder width apart.

Tense your glutes and quads to lock your legs in place.

Contract your inner thigh muscles to try and squeeze the floor between your feet.

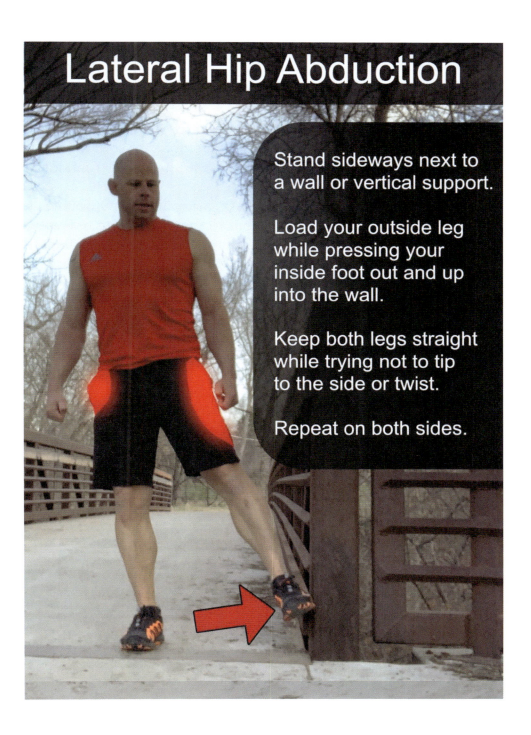

# Standing Twist

Anchor a strap or towel to a sturdy vertical support at about waist height.

Stand sideways with a wide stance and contract your obliques to twist away from the support to apply resistance through the strap.

Maintain an upright posture a repeat on both sides.

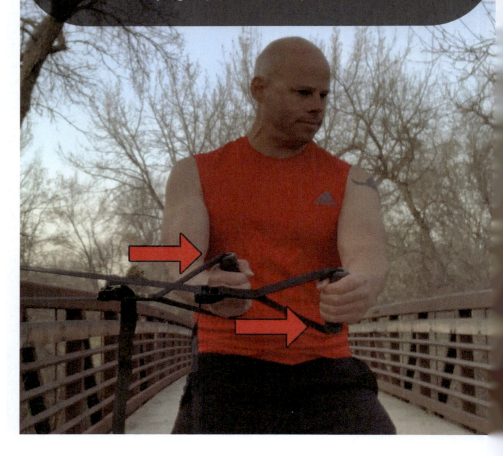

# 8

# Hybrid Isometrics

Isometrics are typically classified into the yielding and overcoming variations. Yielding isometrics involve holding your position against the resistance generated by gravity. Pausing at the top of a pull-up or holding a weight out in front of you are good examples of yielding isometrics. Overcoming isometrics are different because you're creating resistance by pushing or pulling against an unmoving force.

As I mentioned at the beginning of the book, each style has its pros and cons. Yielding isometrics offer a more quantifiable level of resistance, but that resistance is static during the exercise, which may limit the development of either your neural strength or endurance. It can also compromise your neural synergy since it can be more challenging to work on your neural connection and synergy when your goal is only to hold a position for time.

Purely overcoming isometrics isn't always perfect either since the amount of resistance you work with is directly related to your focus and concentration. It can sometimes be challenging to make your muscles work hard enough without any resistance against gravity.

Hybrid isometrics are exercises that are a combination of yielding and overcoming isometrics. It's a variation that places you against the pull of gravity to provide some quantifiable resistance while also using a nylon strap to provide a supplemental source of overcoming resistance.

The exercises in this chapter are a bit more advanced than the techniques in the previous chapters because they either place your body more against gravity or make more use of applying force against a prop like a yoga strap or an iso-loop. The combination of yielding and overcoming resistance can be beneficial for pushing your muscles to a higher level of strength and can help you push beyond the standards you may reach with yielding or overcoming isometrics.

# Hybrid Plank

Loop an iso loop or yoga strap around your lower back and kneel on the ground with the strap under your hands.

Contract your abs and straighten your legs to push your hips up against the strap.

Continue to push hard against the strap while also squeezing the floor together between your hands and feet.

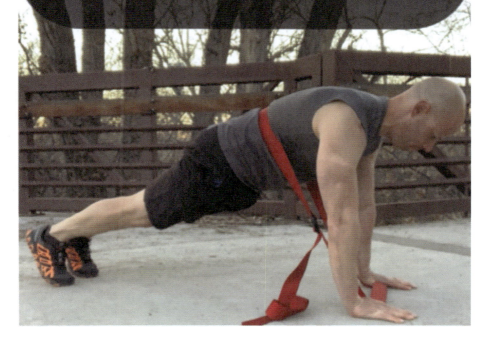

# Hybrid Table Bridge

Sit on the ground with an iso loop or yoga strap around your hips and under your hands.

Drive your heels into the ground to engage your glutes and hamstrings as you lift your hips up against the strap.

Make sure to keep your shoulders down and back as you pull your heels into the ground as if you're trying to pull your feet and hands together.

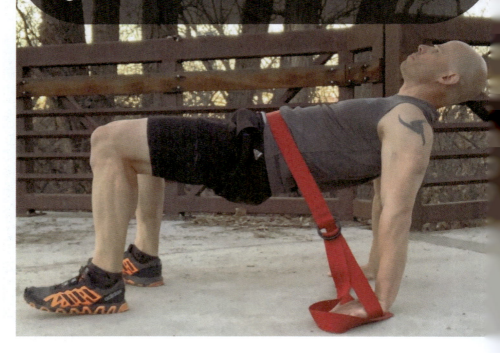

# Hybrid Side Plank

Sit on the ground with the iso loop or yoga strap around your hips and place one hand on the other end of the strap.

Drive the side of your feet and hand into the ground while lifting your hips up sideways against the strap.

Continue to try to squeeze the ground between your hand and foot while keeping your body in a straight line.

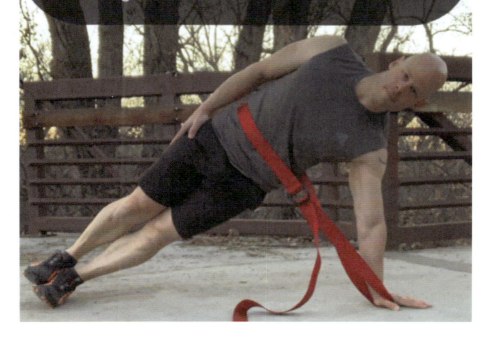

# Hybrid Squat

Run an iso loop or yoga strap under your heels with your feet a little wider than shoulder width apart. Squat down and pull the loop over the upper part of your thighs.

Press hard into your heels as you push your thighs up and outward against the strap.

Keep your weight equally distributed between both the right and left leg.

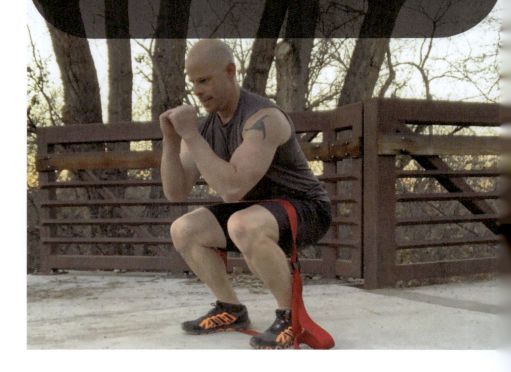

# Hybrid Lunge

Step one foot onto an iso loop or yoga strap and pull the top of the strap over your head to run the strap over the opposite shoulder and around the hips of the front leg.

Shift your hips and front knee forward while keeping your torso upright.

Press into your front heel as you drive your shoulders up against the strap.

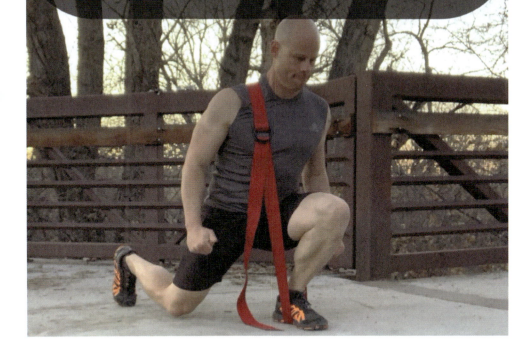

# Hybrid Push-Up

Run an iso loop or yoga strap around your upper back and place your hands on the inside with your elbows bent at a 90 degree angle.

Kneel down and place your hands in a push-ups position on the ground.

Pick your knees up off the ground and press your upper back agains the strap.

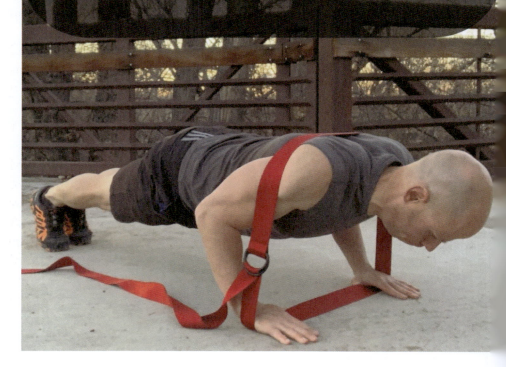

# Hybrid Row

Run a strap across two supports with a suspension device hanging about a foot above the strap.

Place yourself under the strap with the strap near your elbows.

Pull your torso up against the strap and hold with your shoulders down and back.

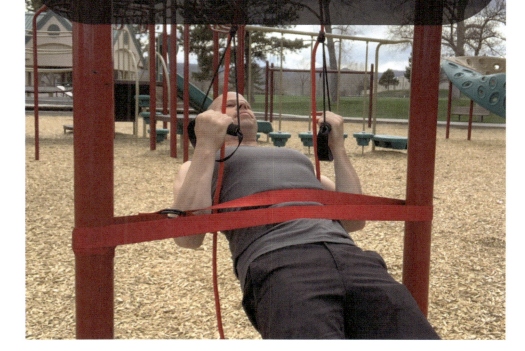

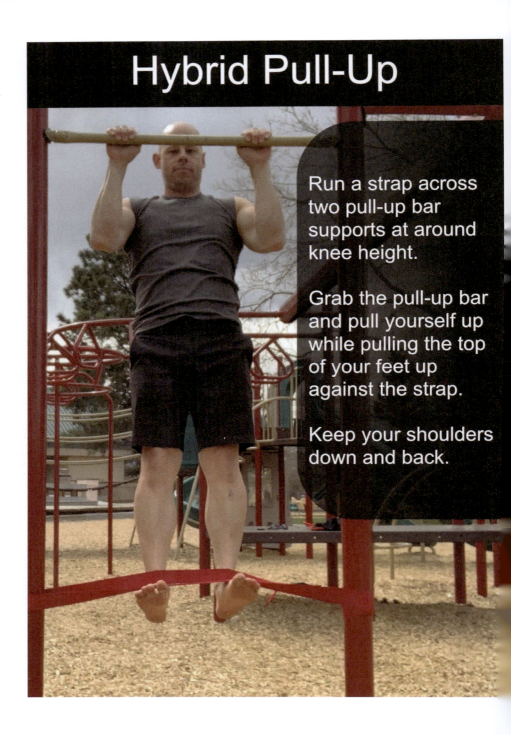

# Hybrid Pull-Up

Run a strap across two pull-up bar supports at around knee height.

Grab the pull-up bar and pull yourself up while pulling the top of your feet up against the strap.

Keep your shoulders down and back.

# 9

# Training Strategies For Success

Overcoming isometrics exercises are a tool, and like any tool, the results you achieve boil down to how well you use these exercises. I don't know the first thing about playing the violin, so I sure wouldn't create anything worth listening to even if you handed me the best violin in the world. The same idea applies to the exercises in this book. They can do wonders for you, but only if you understand how to use them effectively. That's why I wanted to cover some of the most effective strategies for using isometrics in this chapter.

**Start with why**

Any workout or exercise program is only valid if there's a good reason for doing it. You can take the techniques in this book and build a supremely effective plan, but only if you know why you're doing them in the first place. On the other hand, you can do the same techniques, in the same workouts, and end up with nothing but frustration if you lack a compelling purpose behind them. You always want to start designing your overcoming isometric plan around the goals you're setting for yourself. Without that goal, you're like a sailor trying to follow a compass without a needle.

There could be a million reasons for practicing overcoming isometrics, but let's explore a few of the most common goals and how you can best use isometrics to accomplish them.

**Isometrics in solo training**

One of the most common questions I receive is if someone can use isometrics as an effective stand-alone training method.

The simple answer is, of course. You can use any method that can supply tension to your muscles as an effective way to strengthen and condition your muscle tissue. After all, tension is the active ingredient in all forms of training. If there's tension in the muscle, then there's some benefit to doing the exercise.

The other obvious question is if you can achieve the same sort of results with isometrics as you can with classic dynamic training. The clear answer to that is, no, not because one style of exercise is better than the other, but because of the inherently specific nature of all training stimuli.

Every exercise or training method creates an individual neuromuscular pattern, sort of like a neuromuscular fingerprint that can only be created using that very method. So no, you can't accomplish the same results as dynamic training through isometrics. However, you also can't create the same effects of isometric exercise through dynamic exercises either.

The question to ask yourself is if the specific stimulus for one training method is relevant to your goals or not. If your goal involves improving your ability to perform a specific exercise (like push-ups), then yes, you'll need to practice that specific exercise. However, if your goals are less specific, like just building general muscle or strength, then the specifics of one training method over another is less important.

There are several reasons why you may want to practice only isometric training as a strength and conditioning program. You may be curious about how much you can gain from just isometric exercise. You could be looking to take an active break from heavy weight lifting or want to give your joints a break. Overcoming isometric training is also a fantastic travel workout since it requires minimal time, effort, and equipment.

Programing purely isometric workouts are pretty straightforward, especially if you've already been using some sort of a workout routine. All you need to do is use your same workout routine, but convert your dynamic reps into the amount of time you hold an isometric position.

The amount of time it takes to do each rep can vary during a dynamic workout, but generally, one rep takes about 2-3 seconds. So ten reps are going to be roughly 20-30 seconds, and 20 reps are about 40 seconds to one minute. Feel free to adjust and modify these numbers as you like, but if you're used to doing 8-12 reps, then you'll probably feel most comfortable holding an isometric for about 15 seconds. "High rep" training will be around 30-45 seconds and more.

| Isometric Conversion Table | |
|---|---|
| **Dynamic Reps** | **Isometric Time** |
| 5-10 | 10-30 sec. |
| 10-15 | 30-45 sec. |
| 15-20 | 45-60 sec. |

Keep in mind that holding an isometric may feel harder for a given amount of time because you're consistently maintaining a high level of tension in the muscles, so feel free to use slightly less time at first, especially for hybrid isometrics.

**Using isometrics as a warm-up**

Isometrics makes for a fantastic warm-up. The exercises require minimal effort to start doing, which makes them ideal for engaging your mind and body moving when you lack motivation. At the same time, you'll also be priming your neuromuscular system, so you'll be better prepared for more intense exercises later on in the workout.

It's for these reasons that I almost always begin training myself and clients with a quick set of overcoming isometrics.

How you program your isometric warm-up will depend on what you want to accomplish during your workout. If building muscle is your primary objective, you'll want to use the isometrics as both a neural primer as well as a bit of a pre-fatigue technique. This combined stimulus will make it much easier to work your muscles significantly harder during your working sets for muscle growth.

Pre-fatigue isometric workouts can vary in intensity and length, depending on your fitness and skill levels. Doing three sets of an isometric for 10-15 seconds will be an excellent place to start. You can adjust the number of sets and the duration of each set as you see fit. Ideally, you want to be heading into your main workout routine feeling like your muscles have already used up about a third of their available energy.

| Sample Pre-Fatigue Workout | |
|---|---|
| Iso-rows | 15s x 3 |
| Iso-Curls | 15s x 2 |
| Iso- rear fly | 10s x 2 |
| Pull-Ups | 8 x 3 |
| Rows | 15 x 2 |

If your goal is to improve your performance and skills, you'll want to keep your isometric sessions shorter. A shorter contraction will still wake up the muscles you plan on working while helping them stay fresh so you can apply more energy into your actual training. I recommend holding an isometric position for 5-10 seconds for a total of 2-3 rounds or until you feel like you're able to fully engage the muscles you plan on using in your workout.

| Sample Performance Workout | |
| --- | --- |
| Iso-Overhead Press | 10s x 2 |
| Iso- Lateral Raise | 5s x 2 |
| Hand Stand | 20s x 5 |
| Planche | 10s x 3 |

In either case, rest as long as you feel is necessary between your dynamic work sets to be fully ready to put a reasonable effort into your following sets.

**Isometrics during a workout**

Overcoming isometrics is a great supplement within your main workout. The techniques can help you reinforce your neural connections and synergy while also giving your muscles a chance to do more volume with less stress on sensitive joints.

I like to use isometrics within a workout if I feel like I'm having an off day, and my workout feels pretty flat. Including the isometric exercise can boost the intensity of the exercise without using up too much physical or mental energy that may be in short supply.

The best strategy here is to practice an isometric exercise shortly before the dynamic exercise for the same tension chain. That way, you're priming your nervous system before every set to keep your muscles fresh and awake.

| Sample Iso-Dynamic Workout | |
|---|---|
| Hybrid Iso- Squat | 20s |
| Pistol Squat | 8 reps/ leg |
| Hybrid Iso- Squat | 20s |
| Pistol Squat | 8 reps/ leg |
| Hybrid Iso- Squat | 20s |
| Pistol Squat | 8 reps/ leg |

**Isometrics as a finisher**

Isometric training can be a fantastic finishing tool, especially for muscle building workouts, where you're looking to bring your muscles to a very high level of fatigue. They provide you with the perfect opportunity to drive the muscle to a very high level of exhaustion.

Isometric exercises are also a very useful finisher due to the low risk associated with bringing the muscles to such a high level of fatigue. The low risk makes it much easier to push your muscles to the brink of their capabilities without compromising your technique and putting your joints at risk.

| Sample Iso-Finsher Workout | |
|---|---|
| Dips | 12 x 3 |
| Push-Ups | 15 x 2 |
| Iso- Chest Press | 20s x 3 |
| Pressing Chest Fly | 20s x 2 |

The above examples are just that, examples of how you can use the tools of overcoming and hybrid isometrics. These ideas will help you use the exercises in this book to enhance your training proficiency. Ultimately, there is no one best or "correct" way to apply isometric training in your workouts. One of the great things about these techniques is that they are almost impossible to mess up and do incorrectly. So unleash your creativity, experiment, and play around with any ideas that cross your mind. If you feel inspired to use these tools in a new way, I encourage you to roll your sleeves up and just give it a shot. Chances are, it will probably help you discover a new level of your natural potential.

# 10

# Tools Of The Trade

As with calisthenics, overcoming isometrics is a very efficient discipline that requires very little equipment. Many of the techniques don't require any equipment at all, like the chest fly and dead bug. However, picking up a few of the simple tools I mention in this chapter can bring a lot of adjustment and versatility to your training. Most of these tools are pretty inexpensive, and you may already have them lying around the home or gym.

**Iso-Trainer**

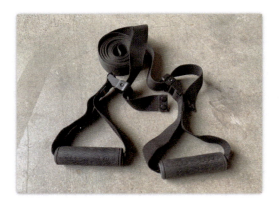

Iso-trainers are a simple length of nylon or a similar strap material with two adjustable handles on each end. The one I'm using in the book comes from a company called WorldFit, and they make a well-made product at a very cost-efficient price.

Iso trainers are very similar in design to many suspension devices, like the gymnastics rings, and some people find they can just use their suspension trainer as a make-shift iso-trainer. I much prefer to have a separate piece of equipment for isometric and suspension workouts, so I don't have to spend the time setting up various exercises.

**Iso-Plate**

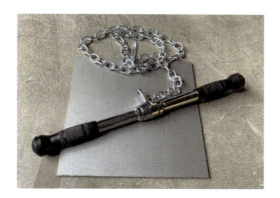

Iso-plates are an old-school isometric tool that allows you to apply a lot of force against a handle that's anchored to a plate you stand on. Commercially available Iso-plates are not the cheapest or most portable isometric training tools. However, they are very sturdy and can be ideal for exercises that require a lot of strength, like iso-deadlifts and squats. That's why a well-made iso-plate can be the ultimate tool for athletes who are looking to apply as much force as possible in an isometric exercise.

## Iso-loop / Yoga strap

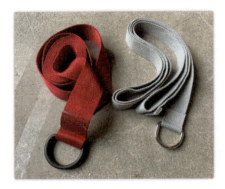

An iso-loop is one of the simplest and most cost-effective isometric training tools you can use. It's nothing more than a single length of nylon strap with a fastener at one end like a cam buckle or set of D-rings. You may already have one of these if you have a set of gymnastics rings or even a simple Yoga strap.

I find it's well worth the cost to purchase a separate piece of equipment for isometric training as opposed to using something you may already be using like gymnastic ring straps. Doing this also has the additional benefit of being able to optimally customize the iso-loop specifically for isometric training.

I order my iso-loops through Strapworks.com, which is one of my all-time favorite companies for such projects. The one I'm using in this book is a 10-foot long nylon strap which is 2-inches wide and has a pair of stainless steel powder-coated D-rings on one end.

The 2-inch wide nylon strap provides the most comfort when pressing against it during hybrid isometrics like the lunge or push-up, which makes it easier to apply more tension in your muscles. I also find the 10-foot length to be long enough for my needs. It's also not so long that I have to hassle with a lot of excess straps material, which is the case with straps from gymnastics rings. The D-rings also make adjusting and tightening down the strap super easy with just one hand, which is very convenient when in an isometric position.

You may find that an 8-foot long strap will be long enough if you're shorter than 5'5" and you may want a 12-foot long strap if you're over 6 feet tall.

**Iso-loop Accessories**

You can expand the versatility of the iso-loop with some of the following attachments, some of which you can find in any commercial gym or home equipment store.

**Towels**

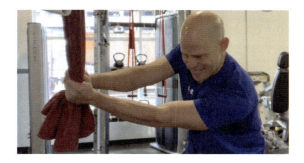

It's amazing what you can do with a simple hand or bath towel. You can use towels to extend the usable range of the iso-loop, provide padding between the strap and your body, use it for a neutral grip, and it helps enhance your isometric grip strength. The set-up is as simple as just folding the towel over the loop and then tightening the loop to the size you need for the exercise.

**Cable attachments**

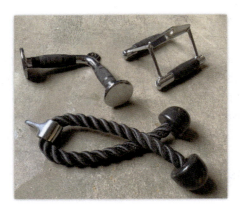

You can use pretty much any cable attachment you find at a local gym with the iso-loop or iso-trainer. Using some of these tools can slightly change the "flavor" of the exercise and might help you discover new ways to wake up a stubborn muscle or two.

# 11

# Frequently Asked Questions

I get a ton of questions regarding isometric training on the Red Delta Project YouTube channel and Instagram. I've done my best to address some of these questions in previous pages, but some of these questions can create a lot of confusion when addressed in long-form. That's why I wrote this special chapter to tackle these questions head-on.

Let's dive in!

**Can you build muscle with isometrics?**

For sure! You can build muscle with any form of training you can use to progress your muscular time under tension. Your time under tension (T.U.T) refers to both the amount of tension in your muscles and the amount of time you're holding that tension for. So essentially, increasing your T.U.T means you progress how hard and long you're working your muscles.

Many people discover that using overcoming isometrics is the key to increasing their T.U.T in both isometric and dynamic exercises. This is partly due to the way overcoming isometrics quickly improves neuromuscular proficiency which is the foundation T.U.T. You may even find you'll place your muscles under more tension and for longer periods of time with overcoming isometrics than you ever could through dynamic training.

**Can Isometrics really help me get stronger?**

Overcoming isometrics can help you build an incredible amount of strength due to the simple fact that strength largely comes from your nervous system.
Overcoming isometrics is first and foremost a neural conditioning method. It directly asks your mind, which controls your nervous system, to make your muscles work. It's because of this, that overcoming isometrics is ideal for helping you build strength by developing it at its neural source.

**Will isometric training help me become a better athlete?**

Absolutely! Overcoming isometrics is all about helping you learn how to use your muscles in a more skillful way. All athletic abilities, from running to swinging a golf club, are about applying tension through your muscles to skillfully perform at a higher level.

Overcoming isometrics won't directly teach you how to improve your jump shot or hold a line on a pair of skis, but it will teach you how to better use the muscles that will help you do those things.

**Are isometrics suitable for beginners?**

I give everyone who's starting out a few isometric exercises to help them get ready for the work ahead of them. Whether they are beginning their training career, a new workout program, or even just a workout, isometrics are the perfect thing to start off with.

**Will isometrics work for older folks?**

Overcoming isometrics are particularly ideal for older individuals or anyone who may have a hard time with dynamic strength training.

Many older adults find they have various injuries or health issues that can make some dynamic forms of exercise a challenge. In addition, years of conforming to poor neuromuscular habits can make dynamic training not only ineffective but also potentially risky.

The gentle intensity of overcoming isometrics means that anyone can begin to educate and work their neuromuscular system to reverse years of neglect or compensation with very little risk to well-worn joints.

**Are isometrics bad if you have high blood pressure?**

Creating, and then holding, a lot of tension can potentially cause a spike in your blood pressure through something called the Valsalva Maneuver. You've probably experienced this action anytime you've lifted something heavy as you held your breath to create more tension in your midsection.

The Valsalva Maneuver is perfectly safe in trained individuals, and it's even an important technique in sports that involve lifting heavy objects. However, it may be undesirable for untrained individuals or people with high blood pressure.

You may find yourself instinctively holding your breath to create more force during isometrics, but this is actually counterproductive to your training. Holding your breath will cause you to fatigue very quickly thus compromising your ability to generate enough force throughout your set. Continuing to breathe throughout the set will not only make the exercise safer, but it will also make it more effective.

**Can I practice Isometrics every day?**

Yep! You can actually practice any sort of exercise you like every day if you like.

Fitness experts often advise you to not practice an exercise every day so you can rest and recover from your training. After all, you don't get results during your exercise, but rather from adapting as you recover after the exercise.

What those same experts often fail to recognize is that you don't have to recover from the actual exercise, but rather from the *fatigue* incurred from the exercise.
While overcoming isometrics typically produces less fatigue than dynamic exercise, it can still be a shock to your system. So let fatigue be your guide. More fatigue requires more rest and vice versa. If you're feeling mentally or physically tired from a training session, then give yourself a day or two. If you're ready to rock and roll, then damn the torpedoes and full speed ahead!

**Will Isometrics help me burn fat?**

Yep! Just as with building muscle and strength, any and all forms of physical activity burn fat through the generation of muscle tension. The more muscle tension you create, and the longer time you generate it for, the more you burn.

Strength training, of any type, not only burns calories while you do it, but there are also powerful carryover effects that make it easier to manage your waistline.

The first is that building stronger muscles makes it easier for you to work longer and harder during other forms of activity. For example, if you're a runner, having stronger legs will make it easier for you to run faster and longer thus helping you burn a lot more calories with less effort.

The second influential carry over is that muscle mass has an influence on your base metabolic rate. There's still some debate over just how much adding a pound of muscle to your frame will help, but it's a sure bet that it will.

## How do I know if I'm making progress in my isometric training?

Your results should be pretty self-evident especially during the first few months of training. You should feel a pretty noticeable improvement in how well you contract your muscles, and how well you can move or work both within and outside of your workouts.

Overcoming isometrics is a great way to rekindle the sensory relationship you have with your body. It's a relationship that's sadly grown dull and rusty for many people due to the neglectful sedentary habits of modern living. If you don't feel like anything is different, it could just be because you're still developing your sensory connection with your muscles.

The other real possibility is that you may very well be in a plateau.

## What do I do when I hit a plateau?

Plateaus are an inevitable part of anyone's training career. Despite the fact that exercise is a potent stimuli for physical change, the fact is the majority of your training career will be spent without a lot of noticeable progress. If it were possible to improve even 1% every week, everyone with a gym membership would become a world class athlete within a few years.

I don't mention this to frustrate you, just to help you understand that fast and noticeable changes will eventually become the exception rather than the norm for you, especially as you mature in your training career.

With that said, your body is always open to receive stimuli it can adapt to. In fact, it's always adapting and changing in one way or another. If you want to create a noticeable change, you have to adjust the stimuli your body is being exposed to. In practical terms, this means changing something in your workout.

You can do this any number of ways from changing how hard you contract a muscle to how long you hold that contraction for. In general, increasing either of those variables will push you along in the direction you want to go in. Just keep in mind that small changes in stimuli typically don't produce large changes in adaptation. Try really ramping things up to break your relative plateau.

If you've been holding an isometric for 15 seconds, try going for a full minute. If you're been going for a minute, go for 15 seconds. Take whatever you consider to be a hard contraction, and try to push or pull twice as hard as you're used to so you double the amount of tension in the muscle.

If either of those objectives seem impossible, then you're on the right track. Always remember, the body only changes when your mind asks it to do something that's just outside of its current range of capability. If you continue to ask your body to do what's it's always done, you'll always end up with the results you currently have.

**What if it feels like the target muscles aren't working?**

Sometimes, achieving that all-important neural connection can be the most difficult step in improving your neural proficiency.

A poor neural connection means your brain isn't really aware there's a muscle there to contract, so it doesn't know how to put tension in it in the first place. It's the physiological case of the blind leading the blind when you're trying to feel a muscle that you can't engage and therefore you can't feel it working.

Overcoming isometrics should eventually overcome this neurological stalemate. All you have to do is continue to try to work the muscle and the signal will eventually grow stronger.

One way you can speed up the process is to look up a visual image of the muscle you're trying to work. Research the origin and insertion points of the muscle so you know where it attaches to your bones as well as the direction the muscle pulls those bones together. Understanding these anatomical facts can help your mind understand just what muscles it's trying to use and how to use them in an effective way.

**How many exercises should you do?**

Probably not as many as you may think. Most of the time, you'll only need to practice one basic compound exercise for each tension chain.
However, feel free to include any of the single joint exercises if you want to target a specific muscle like your hips or shoulder muscles.

I recommend starting out by trying out each of the exercises in this book over the next week or two. Get a feel for each one and how your body responds to it. From there, practice one or two of the exercises in each chain that you can feel work best for you.

**Do I always need to practice overcoming isometrics?**

I always recommend starting out with a couple of basic overcoming isometrics at the start of a workout just to wake up your muscles and make sure they are ready to go.

We are always in a slightly different neural state of awareness due to the natural changes of everyday life. Starting out with a couple of moves is a great way to ensure you're always coming into your workouts with your best neuromuscular foot forward.

With that said, you may reach a point where you feel like your muscles are almost always in an optimal state for training. If that's the case, feel free to cut back on the isometric training but do keep some of the exercises in your routine on a weekly basis.

Your neuromuscular system is in a constant state of change, so you never know what new habits or imbalances you are currently developing. Practicing a few basic techniques once or twice a week can help prevent such imbalances and poor habits from developing.

**Conclusion**

Well, my friend, you've reached the end of the book, but your isometric journey is just beginning.
I'm very excited for you to experience the benefits of this super-efficient training discipline, so please make a promise to yourself to start putting what you've learned here into practice asap. Don't wait until Monday, or for that new project at work to wrap up. Take action as soon as you can so you can be well on your way to stronger, safer, and more satisfying workouts.

I invite you to also continue your training journey through the Red Delta Project YouTube Channel, where I have an entire video playlist dedicated to overcoming isometric training. I also have plenty more for you to discover over at reddeltaproject.com as well. As always, feel free to reach out to me at reddeltaproject@gmail.com with any questions you may have. I would also love to hear about your success and accomplishments, as well.

Be fit, live free,
Matt Schifferle

# About the Author

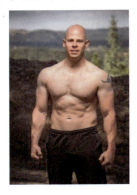

Matt Schifferle is the founder of the Red Delta Project, an online resource dedicated to helping you maximize your results through minimalist fitness strategies.

You can learn more at **https://www.reddeltaproject.com** and discover more on the Red Delta Project YouTube channel. You can also search for the Red Delta Project Podcast in your favorite podcast directory.

Feel free to reach out to Matt through email (**reddeltaproject@gmail.com**) or you can DM him on Instagram @red.delta.project.

Look for these other R.D.P titles, in paperback and Kindle format on Amazon:

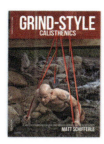
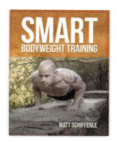
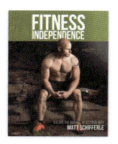
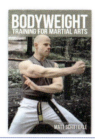
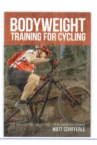
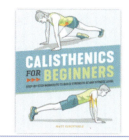

Printed in Great Britain
by Amazon